Acceptance and Commitment Therapy and Brain Injury

Acceptance and Commitment Therapy and Brain Injury discusses how acceptance and commitment therapy (ACT) can be integrated into existing approaches to neuropsychological rehabilitation and therapy used with people who have experienced a brain injury.

Written by practising clinical psychologists and clinical neuropsychologists, this text is the first to integrate available research with innovative clinical practice. The book discusses how ACT principles can be adapted to meet the broad and varying physical, cognitive, emotional and behavioural needs of people who have experienced brain injury, including supporting families of people who have experienced brain injury and healthcare professionals working in brain injury services. It offers considerations for direct and indirect, systemic and multidisciplinary working through discussion of ACT concepts alongside examples taken from clinical practice and consideration of real-world brain injury cases, across a range of clinical settings and contexts.

The book will be relevant to a range of psychologists and related professionals, including those working in neuropsychology settings and those working in more general physical or mental health contexts.

Dr Will Curvis is a Clinical Psychologist in the NHS, working mainly in acute inpatient physical health and neuropsychology services with people with long-term physical health problems and neurological conditions. He also works as a Clinical Tutor for the Doctorate in Clinical Psychology programme at Lancaster University.

Dr Abigail Methley is a Clinical Psychologist in the NHS supporting people with neurological conditions in an outpatient neuropsychology service. In her independent practice she supports people recovering from trauma and living with neurodiversity. She is a clinical researcher and publishes regularly on mental health and neuropsychology practice issues.

"This is a helpful book for practitioners and researchers alike. Acceptance and commitment therapy is becoming more widely known and researched within the field of neurological conditions and a book aimed at working with people with brain injury and their families and systems is a timely addition to the literature."

Fiona Eccles, Clinical Psychologist and Lecturer, Lancaster University

"Will Curvis and Abigail Methley are to be congratulated for this timely collation of relevant research and practical guidance on ACT, showing how the approach can be used to support psychological wellbeing in people with neurological conditions. Particular highlights are scene-setting from experts by experience and discussion of cultural considerations, together with insights into the use of ACT with specific brain injury presentations in a variety of settings."

Katherine Carpenter, Consultant Clinical Neuropsychologist and Chair of The British Psychological Society's Division of Neuropsychology

"This really is an excellent compendium of chapters which most helpfully detail the potential for acceptance and commitment therapy to improve the psychological well-being of people with a range of different neurological conditions. I particularly valued the chapter on progressive neurological conditions given the relative lack of therapeutic approaches currently available for this group of individuals."

Jane Simpson, Professor of the Psychology of Neurodegenerative Conditions, Lancaster University

"This is a much-needed book. ACT is a well-established psychological therapy but there have been very few comprehensive accounts of how ACT can be used to support people in the context of brain injury. This book illustrates very practically how ACT can be integrated into holistic neuropsychological rehabilitation, with both adults and children, in a wide range of neurological conditions. Importantly, the book discusses how ACT can be adapted for people with moderate or severe brain injury, whilst retaining its core focus on committed action, being present and values-based goal setting. There is something for everyone in this book – whether you are new to ACT, new to neuropsychological rehabilitation or an old hand at both, this book will be useful."

Jon Evans, Professor of Applied Neuropsychology, Institute of Health and Wellbeing, University of Glasgow

"Neuropsychologists working in brain injury rehabilitation will want to read this book about ACT as most survivors of stroke, traumatic brain injury, encephalitis, anoxia and other diagnoses will have both cognitive and emotional problems. For the emotional problems, ACT has become an important tool and this edited book will provide a wealth of detailed information addressing a range of related topics including mild and severe injury, cultural issues, identity, holistic rehabilitation, future directions and the concerns of both adults and children."

Barbara A. Wilson, OBE, Clinical Neuropsychologist and
Honorary Professor at the University of Hong Kong, the
University of Sydney and the University of East Anglia

Acceptance and Commitment Therapy and Brain Injury

A Practical Guide for Clinicians

Edited by Will Curvis
and Abigail Methley

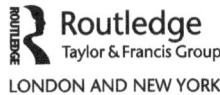 Routledge
Taylor & Francis Group

LONDON AND NEW YORK

First published 2022
by Routledge
2 Park Square, Milton Park, Abingdon, Oxon OX14 4RN

and by Routledge
605 Third Avenue, New York, NY 10158

Routledge is an imprint of the Taylor & Francis Group, an informa business

British Library Cataloguing-in-Publication Data
A catalogue record for this book is available from the British Library

Library of Congress Cataloging-in-Publication Data
Names: Curvis, Will, editor. | Methley, Abigail, editor.
Title: Acceptance and commitment therapy and brain injury: a practical guide for clinicians / edited by Will Curvis and Abigail Methley.
Description: Milton Park, Abingdon, Oxon; New York, NY: Routledge, 2022. | Includes bibliographical references and index.
Identifiers: LCCN 2021027738 (print) | LCCN 2021027739 (ebook) | ISBN 9780367456313 (hardback) | ISBN 9780367456245 (paperback) | ISBN: 9781003024408 (ebook)
Subjects: LCSH: Brain damage–Treatment. | Acceptance and commitment therapy.
Classification: LCC RC387.5 .A272 2022 (print) | LCC RC387.5 (ebook) | DDC 617.4/81044–dc23
LC record available at https://lccn.loc.gov/2021027738
LC ebook record available at https://lccn.loc.gov/2021027739

ISBN: 9780367456313 (hbk)
ISBN: 9780367456245 (pbk)
ISBN: 9781003024408 (ebk)

DOI: 10.4324/9781003024408

Typeset in Times New Roman
by Newgen Publishing UK

This book is dedicated to the people whose stories and experiences have inspired this book – everyone who has experienced a brain injury or lives with a neurological condition and their loved ones. Any financial proceeds from this book will be donated to Headway – the brain injury charity based in the UK (registered charity 1025852), as a small gesture of gratitude for their enduring work in providing support, information and advocacy to people who have experienced brain injury.

Contents

Foreword

Ray Owen

Most creatures, most of the time, have an overwhelming urge to survive. If our own survival, or that of someone who matters to us, is seriously threatened – by something like an acquired brain injury (ABI) – then living past that immediate danger is understandably a cause for celebration. Sometimes the immediate recovery and rehabilitation period after the damage of the injury or the necessary treatment sees improvements that bring relief, reward and hope for a speedy return to the life that was being lived before the event, and the kind of future we wanted.

Sometimes that's the outcome people get.

And often it isn't.

There may be limited recovery, or even with great strides there may be residual limitations: poorer concentration and memory than before, difficulty with planning, being more emotionally reactive, significant fatigue, struggling with loud noise or complex environments. There are knock-on effects for that "normal" life we were hoping to get back to – there may be an impact on your ability to do your previous job, on your family life, or your leisure pursuits.

There may be an impact on a person's view of themselves, their world and their future. They will have to deal with difficult thoughts and feelings that any rational person might have under such circumstances. It is no surprise that periods of low mood, frustration and anger, and fear of the future are common. Whether or not accompanied by suicidal thoughts, some will ask whether this "new" life is actually a life worth living.

Many of these challenges are not unique to ABI. Long-term physical health problems – ones which are not amenable to cure, so will be a presence in the person's life for the foreseeable future – often challenge our ability to live well. Think of chronic pain, diabetes, serious lung or heart conditions, bowel disorders, multiple sclerosis. In the UK, around one in five people is living with such a condition, and that figure rises to 58% in the over-60s (Department of Health, 2012). While the precise pattern of physical symptoms, impairment and treatment burden can vary greatly between different conditions, some symptoms are present in many (pain, fatigue, reduced mobility), and common themes around the implications for quality of life are often seen.

Can I continue to work? How can I be a good parent if I can't provide, or play actively with my child? Where's the fun in life if I can't run / dance / garden / sing any more? How can I plan anything if I'm not sure what I can manage later today, tomorrow, next month or next year?

No wonder the condition feels like an enemy that has taken over our lives. For sure, there are sometimes "silver linings" – changes in life priorities, new insights into relationships or beneficial changes of direction. However, for the most part, we have to acknowledge the pain and loss that a long-term health condition brings.

It is understandable to treat a long-term condition such as a brain injury as an enemy to be fought against, something to be overcome in order to regain one's old self. But that is often a victory that cannot be achieved. Losing oneself in an unending, unwinnable battle against this aspect of yourself can actively prevent finding a different way of living well under these new circumstances.

One benefit of conceptualising life after an ABI as being like living with other types of long-term physical health conditions is the possibility that knowledge, skills and experience gained in helping people adjust successfully and find ways of living well with health conditions may also be useful (in whole or in part) for helping people adjust and cope after a brain injury.

There are many ways of supporting people in these situations. One of those is the Psychological Flexibility approach – more formally termed Contextual Behavioural Science, but most widely known in the form of acceptance and commitment therapy (ACT; Hayes et al., 1999).

This contemporary form of behaviour therapy – with over 300 randomised controlled trials published in peer-reviewed journals – directly addresses many of the challenges described above: how do we move towards the kind of life that brings us fulfilment? How do we deal with difficult thoughts and feelings that inevitably show up along the way? In particular, what can we do about all those unhelpful habits we humans commonly fall into – getting hooked by thoughts – especially critical ones, worrying about the future or avoiding important things because of how bad they make us feel? These are questions that can be applied to all areas of human life, from traditional mental health domains, through addictions, education, relationship-managing stigma, shame and workplace stress, organisational and societal change, amongst others. Crucially, since its earliest days, ACT has been applied to working with people with long-term physical health problems, in both group and individual settings.

But how can one therapeutic approach hope to be effective across such a range of difficulties? The ACT approach proposes a set of common human responses to the experiences of life that can help us understand how we get stuck and help us move forward. Those same processes are seen to apply in lots of different contexts; though exactly how they play out, and how best we can help shift them, will of course depend on the details of that situation. Therefore, we can say we are dealing with *universal processes in specific contexts*. While there are many excellent books explaining the ACT model, a book like this one will help you understand its application to this specific context of working with people who have experienced a brain injury.

Dealing with universal processes, the ACT approach is equally applicable to the person with the health condition, to a family member or indeed to a health professional seeking to support them. Each person has their own set of values that they live by; each person takes actions that move them towards or further away from those values; and each person has particular ways of dealing with unwanted thoughts and feelings that show up as they do that. The best outcome for the person with the ABI will involve understanding and support for all of the people around them. It can be useful to have a common framework for understanding, to help with the problems each person is facing from their own perspective.

In this book you will have the opportunity to consider how ACT can be applied to work with people with brain injuries and neurological conditions of different kinds and of different levels of severity, to support adjustment, coping and wellbeing. You will also read about how ACT concepts can be applied within different contexts and to work with different groups of people, including with children, with families and with healthcare staff themselves.

There's a saying in the ACT community: "A life well lived is a life lived according to your values". Existence throws up barriers to that – and ABI can certainly bring about some extra challenges. This book will help you learn about ways of helping people deal better with those challenges, to support people to go beyond simply surviving their brain injury and to go on to live a fulfilling life in its presence.

References

Department of Health. (2012). Long term conditions compendium of information (3rd ed.). https://assets.publishing.service.gov.uk/government/uploads/system/uploads/attachment_data/file/216528/dh_134486.pdf

Hayes, S. C., Strosahl, K. D., & Wilson, K. G. (1999). *Acceptance and commitment therapy: An experiential approach to behavior change.* Guilford Press.

Preface

Will Curvis and Abigail Methley

A brain injury can happen to anyone, at any time. In the UK, someone has a brain injury about every 90 seconds. An ever-increasing body of research literature and clinical guidelines – alongside work by charities and patient-led organisations – highlights the importance of neuropsychologically informed approaches to recovery and wellbeing following brain injury, considering the physical, emotional, cognitive and functional consequences that a brain injury can have on people's lives.

However traditional goal-orientated psychological therapies such as cognitive-behavioural therapy, which focus on symptom reduction and are generally specific to particular diagnostic categories such as depression or anxiety, often struggle to meet the needs of people with brain injuries. The enduring physical, behavioural, cognitive and emotional changes or impairments that brain injury can cause may act as a barrier to this kind of therapeutic approach. An emphasis on changing or shifting negative thoughts is difficult when those thoughts are valid and powerful. Increasing levels of positive activity and working towards goals can feel overwhelming for a person who can no longer do the things they used to.

Conversely, more exploratory or open-ended approaches such as psychodynamic psychotherapy or person-centred counselling can lack the direction or focus on behavioural change that people with brain injuries are often seeking. And at the other end of the spectrum, neuropsychological rehabilitation that does not pay attention to the emotional components (e.g. being overly focused on compensatory strategies or restoration of cognitive ability) can feel cold and disconnected. We are our brains, and our brains are us – a brain injury can change the whole essence of who we are and can fundamentally affect how we live our lives. A therapeutic approach that lacks *feeling* is missing something very fundamental.

Acceptance and commitment therapy (ACT; pronounced as a word, not an acronym) has emerged as a popular approach to psychological therapy, amongst a range of other "third-wave" therapies which emphasise the value of meta-cognition, mindfulness, emotions, acceptance and values – as well as the processes intrinsic to the therapeutic relationship.

Relational Frame Theory, upon which ACT is based, proposes that developing verbal language through relating constructs and concepts can have some unfortunate downsides. We can experience pain and distress as a result of thoughts or worries that may never happen, and we can become trapped by cycles of negative rumination and regret. Through our memories, mental images, emotions, sensations and urges, our lives are governed by how we *think*. We are hard-wired to attend to these mental experiences, often at the cost of becoming disconnected from the direct experience of the world around us. Trying not to think about these difficult thoughts often inadvertently causes us to think about them more.

ACT approaches therefore encourage us to improve our "psychological flexibility" – if we can learn to experience events, feelings, thoughts and sensations as unpleasant but transient, we can change our relationship with them. Instead of being caught up in those unpleasant thoughts, feelings and sensations (or our efforts to try to change or avoid them), we can just let them simply exist – then get on with living our lives in a way which connects to what is most important to us.

As an approach to psychological therapy, ACT focuses on universal processes to support psychological flexibility, applied in a transdiagnostic way. ACT does not seek to change or challenge unpleasant thoughts or feelings; rather, ACT aims to help us to become more aware of how our reactions to thoughts and feelings can interfere with living the life we want to live, according to our values. We like how Russ Harris (2019) simplifies psychological flexibility into three core processes – *be present, open up* and *do what matters*.

In the context of brain injury, ACT offers a powerful alternative to other therapeutic modalities. ACT is about committed behavioural change; it is about making positive improvements in life, guided by and in line with values. It is also about learning to conceptualise and cope with difficult thoughts, feelings and sensations in a more flexible and compassionate way. As a result, ACT has become increasingly popular as a therapeutic approach to supporting people to cope with or adjust to emotional, difficult and overwhelming situations – such as living with a long-term physical health condition, chronic pain or life-limiting disability. We believe these foundations and guiding principles make ACT a valuable approach to consider when working with people who have experienced brain injury.

Written by practising clinical psychologists and clinical neuropsychologists, this text is the first to integrate the available research with innovative clinical practice to consider how ACT might be used with people who have experienced a brain injury. *Part I* discusses how ACT might fit alongside or be incorporated into neuropsychological approaches to therapy and rehabilitation following brain injury, in terms of supporting coping, adjustment and psychological wellbeing.

While there are many excellent books explaining the ACT approach, learning about and practising ACT are more difficult when working with people with complex physical, cognitive and emotional problems. Therefore, *Part II* considers how ACT principles might be adapted to meet the needs of a range of specific populations within this broad definition of brain injury – including working with children or adults with mild, moderate and severe brain injuries. We discuss other kinds of brain damage such as that caused by progressive neurological conditions, alongside considerations around using ACT-based approaches across different cultural contexts. This section is not an exhaustive list of every possible presentation, symptom or variable that practitioners might encounter when working in brain injury services. It is also not a deep dive into the theoretical or philosophical underpinnings of ACT. We hope that it is a practical guide which illustrates the breadth and transferability of ACT principles, supporting clinicians to think creatively about how they might adapt their approach to meet the unique and individual needs of the people they work with.

In *Part III*, we step back and think more broadly about how ACT principles might be applied and transferred flexibly across different contexts, in order to support the needs of people who have experienced brain injury. We discuss how ACT ideas might be delivered via peer-support groups, or adapted to work with families. We consider how ACT principles might contribute towards systemic change within brain injury services, drawing on examples from work in homelessness services. As above, we do not intend this to be exhaustive or the final word on this topic – we hope that this section will inspire aspiring, trainee and qualified psychological professionals to have wider conversations about how ACT ideas and principles might be further adapted, integrated and applied to support people across other clinical settings and contexts.

In developing this book, we stand on the shoulders of giants. All the chapters in this text seek to build on work from other key authors, particularly in the fields of ACT and neuropsychological rehabilitation (some key introductory texts are recommended below). We are indebted to everyone within the neuropsychology, ACT and contextual behavioural science communities for helping to shape our thinking – we have referenced and credited ideas wherever possible but recognise that the collaborative nature of these communities has been key in how work in these fields has developed. We would like to give our heartfelt thanks to the clinicians and writers who have served as inspiration for this book, including everyone who has written a book or paper, or contributed via social media (e.g. on Twitter or in the various Facebook networks, such as the "Neuro-ACT" or "Acceptance and Commitment Therapy for Practitioners" groups).

Above all else, this book has been inspired by the stories and experiences of the people that we have worked with and their families. Although most of the clinical work described in the book is anonymised, with details changed to protect confidentiality, we are eternally grateful to the people who have contributed to the development of this work by being willing to talk about values, eat raisins mindfully and sing their negative thoughts to the tunes of power ballads from the 80s. We hope you enjoy it.

Suggested further reading

Acceptance and commitment therapy

Bennett, R., & Oliver, J. (2019). *Acceptance and commitment therapy: 100 Key points & techniques*. Routledge.

Hayes, S., Strosahl, K. D., & Wilson, K. G. (2011). *Acceptance and commitment therapy: The process and practice of mindful change*. Guilford Press.

Brain injury and neuropsychological rehabilitation

Newby, G., Coetzer, R., Daisley, A., & Weatherhead, S. (2013). *Practical neuropsychological rehabilitation in acquired brain injury: A guide for working clinicians*. Routledge.

Törneke, N. (2010). *Learning RFT: An introduction to relational frame theory and its clinical application*. New Harbinger.

Wilson, B., Gracey, F., Evans, J., & Bateman, A. (2009). *Neuropsychological rehabilitation: Theory, models, therapy and outcome*. Cambridge University Press.

ACT and brain injury

Kangas, M., & McDonald, S. (2011). Is it time to act? The potential of acceptance and commitment therapy for psychological problems following acquired brain injury. *Neuropsychological Rehabilitation*, 21(2), 250–276. https://doi.org/10.1080/09602011.2010.540920

Todd, D., & Smith, M. (2019). Acceptance and commitment therapy (ACT) after brain injury. In: G. Yeates, & F. Ashworth (Eds.), *Psychological therapies in acquired brain injury* (pp. 132–153). Routledge.

Whiting, D. L., Simpson, G. K., Ciarrochi, J., & McLeod, H. J. (2012). Assessing the feasibility of acceptance and commitment therapy in promoting psychological adjustment after severe traumatic brain injury. *Brain Injury, 26*(4–5), 588–589. https://doi.org/10.1017/brimp.2012.28

Reference

Harris, R. (2019). *ACT made simple* (2nd ed.). New Harbinger.

Part I

Introducing ACT and brain injury

Chapter 1

Setting the scene

The impact of brain injury

Harriet Holmes, Paul Twist and Holly

My story: Harriet Holmes

In the early hours of Easter Sunday 2018, my mum was rushed to hospital for lifesaving surgery to repair an aortic dissection. She remained in a coma in intensive care for 17 days, during which time CT scans showed that she had suffered a number of strokes during the initial surgery. Once stable, she was transferred to the acute stroke unit, where she spent 2 months regaining skills like walking, communicating, feeding and basic self-care. The pain of seeing her like this was unimaginable – we felt hopeless and exhausted and survival mode seemed to kick in to get us through. Life as we knew it had changed and the future felt terrifying and uncertain.

Two years on and after a lengthy neurorehabilitation process, our family is thankfully in a very different place. Recovery has brought its own challenges and there have been many painful adjustments for each of us along the way.

The hardest part for me, as her daughter, is the sense of loss, despite her still being here. Others seem to struggle to understand this in the context of her recovery, which can leave me feeling guilty, alone and ungrateful for the fact she survived. As her level of insight increased, I worried how she would adjust and how the cognitive and physical impacts of the strokes would affect her emotionally. The brain injury led to significant fatigue and breathing complications, requiring further surgery, meaning physical exercise has been incredibly difficult for her. Being unable to return to driving quickly and unable to engage in the activities she loves (including ballroom dancing) has caused her considerable distress. More subtle skills like planning, organising and executing tasks can still be difficult for her when she is tired. Mum found it helpful to speak with the Clinical Psychologist within her rehab team about managing the expectations she placed on her brain and body to perform as she had pre-injury.

As an Assistant Psychologist myself working within the field of neuro-disability, I have found my role incredibly challenging both personally and professionally since this happened. Managing the daily triggers, the worries

DOI: 10.4324/9781003024408-2

about the impact on my career and the emotional toll of working with families who are going through similar experiences has felt impossible at times. Accessing my own support to process the initial trauma and reflect on the ongoing impact has been lifechanging.

When something like this happens, it makes you realise and reconnect with what's important and gives a sense of perspective. Whilst I fully appreciate the long-term emotional impact that brain injury can have on families, I am starting to acknowledge some "positives" that my mum's brain injury has brought; for example, learning to focus on the present. Mum embraced her early medical retirement from her career in academia, which gives her the time to focus on her recovery and the things important to her. Although new and unexpected challenges have arisen at each stage and transition, our family has survived – despite each coping in very different ways. The critical period drew us together physically, but over time, we are learning how to communicate and support each other more effectively. It feels more important than ever to be close to home, family and valued relationships.

Don't strokes only happen to old people?: Paul Twist

I'm Paul and my brain injury was the result of a haemorrhagic stroke I had in March 2014 at the age of 35. The stroke hit me suddenly one afternoon at work. I still remember the stroke happening. I was eating a chocolate bar containing peanuts and wondered if my face was going numb due to an undiagnosed nut allergy. I then went into a meeting and recall my manager seeming concerned. However, my primary worry at the time was that I wouldn't be able to go to the pub after work that evening. Little did I realise that the changes to my life would be considerably more significant!

In the long term, the greatest impact my brain injury has had on me has definitely been physical. I am no longer able to use my left limbs functionally, which means I have to use a powered wheelchair to get around. This impairment of my mobility has led to significant loss of independence, which I have struggled with somewhat as I am no longer able to do whatever I like whenever I like. This means I am less able to use public transport, which therefore means I can no longer go to gigs by myself (as a big indie and punk fan, this was a huge part of my life before the stroke). Even simple everyday things that one takes for granted, such as sitting on the sofa if I'm home alone, I am wary of doing now as I'm unable to get back into my wheelchair quickly enough to answer the door.

Also, having to rely on others for assistance with some basic everyday tasks such as getting dressed can make me feel rather useless, as well as feeling guilty for the imposition on my wife, who has been extraordinarily helpful ever since the brain injury occurred. I have also noticed that following my brain injury, I have become more anxious. I was always a rather anxious person, but my anxiety levels have increased to the point where, even 5 years down the road of recovery, I still feel some anxiety upon leaving my home, even if it's just to make my way to the local shop in my wheelchair. This is because I worry about losing control of my wheelchair and drifting into the road. I also seem to cry at the drop of a hat (perhaps literally, if it's a nice hat and it's been damaged by being dropped). I suppose in a nutshell, following the brain injury, my emotional responses have been heightened. So, if I was easily stressed and emotional prior to the stroke, this has been greatly amplified post-stroke.

A phrase my wife has caught me exclaiming on more than one occasion is "I'm sick of everything!" And while this is melodramatic hyperbole rather than a reflection of my actual state of mind, it's perhaps a useful insight into how I often feel overwhelmed following my brain injury.

Day zero: Holly

Backwards

Day zero. 17 February 2017.
Hit by a speeding car (52 mph), broken bones, diffuse axonal brain injury.
A soporific, choking cloud descends. The Great Depression.
Loss on loss on loss on loss. I lose all sense of myself.
The once confident, healthy, quick-witted joker.
Gone.
Replaced, displaced, by a clumsy, sluggish, emotional wrecking ball.
I am such a disappointment.
Flailing for control, I refuse to accept this state is forever.
Embarrassed apologies, scribbled reminders on neon Post-It notes, calendar
    entries, alarms.
Public red-hot shame.
Spontaneous acts of audacious courage, desperate to catch a glimpse of the
    old me in others' eyes. I cling like a limpet to my former sense of self.
I win a cycling race 2 months after the accident, with a still broken tibia. For
    a fleeting, euphoric moment. I am me again! Then, back.
Thudding to earth,
Unable to recall my age when interviewed by the local press.
I am such a disappointment.
I stubbornly continue grappling with Old Man Time, arms outstretched into
    the past.
Fingertips temptingly brushing through my shadow. A shimmering ghost of
    the person I achingly need back. But who died that day.
I'm right there, fingers so frustratingly close.
Just lean in, a bit more … Come on!

Forwards

Day zero. 17 February 2017.

Hit by a speeding car (52 mph), broken bones, diffuse axonal brain injury.

A soporific, choking cloud descended. Lost, distraught searching. That cloud still looms occasionally. A heavy shadow. But there is more sunlight now.

Slivers of silver strands of sunshine burst through unexpectedly, catching me off guard.

Small moments of clarity. Sharp realisations of a life still of value. Overwhelming appreciation. Deep, enveloping gratitude. Acknowledged love.

A weighted blanket soothing me.

I will be OK.

Often I see a blank page ahead, waiting to be written. The future is the only thing I can control. It seems fresh and clean and exciting. Infinite possibility, eagerly waiting to be scribed.

I push forwards. Upwards. I have narrowly escaped death – how else can I behave? Everything that came before had to happen for us to be the person we are now, and the greatest moments of clarity come when we look back and realise it was all necessary and all beautiful.

Life is not perfect. I am not who I was, nor will I ever be. But I might again feel clean and bright.

My future self shimmers. Just out of reach.

Just lean in, a bit more … Come on!

Chapter 2

Integrating acceptance and commitment therapy into holistic neuropsychological rehabilitation

Victoria Teggart, Cara Thompson and Thomas Rozwaha

Abstract

Acceptance and commitment therapy (ACT) draws on psychological theories of human language and behaviour to help people navigate difficult life events. ACT encourages the development of "psychological flexibility" to support people to navigate life's challenges and live a meaningful life, even in the presence of difficult thoughts and feelings. Neuropsychological rehabilitation draws on a range of theories and techniques to support people after a brain injury. ACT principles can be weaved into a neurorehabilitation framework to provide a person-centred, values-based approach.

Someone is admitted to hospital with a brain injury every 3 minutes, with many experiencing varied and lifelong difficulties following their injury. Changes in ability and well-being can have a profound impact on a person's life. Acquired brain injury (ABI) is a term used to describe rapid-onset brain injury of any cause, such as those caused by stroke, traumatic injury or infection. The brain injury association Headway (2019) reported that 348,453 people were admitted into hospital in the UK with an ABI in 2016–2017, equating to the occurrence of a brain injury every 3 minutes. After a brain injury, many people access specialist neuropsychological rehabilitation, an approach rooted in behavioural psychology, cognitive neuropsychology and psychotherapy. Neuropsychological rehabilitation aims to facilitate adjustment, increase independence and improve quality of life.

ABI can lead to a broad range of consequences, which impact the individual, their family and the systems that surround them (Royal College of Physicians & British Society of Rehabilitation Medicine, 2003). Common difficulties experienced following brain injury can include, but are not limited to:

- Changes in physical mobility
- Chronic pain
- Fatigue

DOI: 10.4324/9781003024408-3

- Cognitive deficits such as reduced concentration, poor memory and difficulties with planning or ability to problem solve
- Difficulties with behavioural regulation that may result in the presence of challenging behaviour, apathy or reduced motivation
- High levels of emotional distress as a reaction to the brain injury and its consequences
- Changes in ability to regulate emotions
- Reduced awareness of, or insight into, the changes resulting from the brain injury
- Feelings of loss and grief
- Changes in sense of self or identity.

Changes in abilities and emotional well-being often have a negative impact on an individual's life circumstances, such as loss of valued roles, difficulties with employment and strains on relationships (Whiting et al., 2019). Rehabilitation and recovery following brain injury can involve a long journey of adjustment to changes in ability as well as finding new meaning in life (Freeman et al., 2015).

Neuropsychological rehabilitation following ABI

Many who experience ABI are able to access some form of rehabilitation, which might be during the early phase of their illness in hospital, in specialised neurorehabilitation settings or in the community following discharge from acute hospital care. Best practice for brain injury rehabilitation requires involvement of a range of health and social care professionals (National Institute for Health and Care Excellence (NICE), 2014).

Neuropsychological rehabilitation refers to any strategies or techniques aimed at supporting people with cognitive, emotional and behavioural changes experienced following ABI. As outlined above, these difficulties are wide-ranging and not easily separable into single problems to target (Wilson, 2017). Neuropsychological rehabilitation can be viewed as a process aimed at increasing independence and facilitating adjustment to all of the consequences of brain injury (Jackson & Hague, 2013).

Given the scope of neuropsychological problems that can arise following ABI, holistic neuropsychological rehabilitation draws on a range of psychological theories and approaches in order to meet the complex needs of these individuals. New approaches have been incorporated into neuropsychological rehabilitation over time, to include advances in understanding of neuropsychological difficulties and the evolution of intervention strategies.

Significant contributions to the practice of neuropsychological rehabilitation have been drawn from:

- Cognitive neuropsychology: to provide an understanding of cognitive functioning, leading to the development of approaches to assess cognitive strengths and weaknesses and techniques to support individuals in either relearning skills or compensating for deficits.
- Behavioural psychology: which has provided the foundation for many neuropsychological rehabilitation programmes (Wilson, 2017). Behavioural theories are useful in understanding why people respond in certain ways, how internal and external events contribute to responses and how people can be supported to change their behaviour.
- A wide range of psychotherapeutic traditions: psychoanalysis, psychodynamic therapy, cognitive-behavioural therapy and cognitive analytic therapy have been variously applied to the understanding of emotional difficulties following brain injury (Weatherhead et al., 2013). Whilst all of these approaches have demonstrated benefit, no single method or technique has been found to address all difficulties for all individuals.

As neuropsychological rehabilitation has evolved over time, it is important to consider how new and innovative psychological approaches may be applied, in continuing to meet the needs of those who have experienced ABI.

Acceptance and commitment therapy

Life is full of both positive and challenging experiences. While some experiences are hoped for, or even expected, some show up whether they are wanted or not. Nevertheless, those experiences contribute to what it is to be human – and life is tough to navigate. Acceptance and commitment therapy (ACT) is an approach which focuses on living with these experiences and changing responses to painful thoughts and feelings, in the service of working towards living a meaningful and value-based life (Hayes et al., 2006).

ACT is made up of a set of principles which have in common the underlying idea that life is a "process to be lived, not a problem to be solved" (Hayes, 2019, p. 10). The ACT philosophy attempts to empower people by shifting attention to what matters in life. Further, ACT ideas promote action guided by core values, awareness and willingness to experience and engage (Harris, 2019). As such, ACT can be used as a therapeutic approach for people experiencing a range of difficulties and distress, without requiring someone's difficulties to fit into a particular psychiatric diagnostic category (Dindo et al., 2017).

One of the strengths of ACT is its grounding in well-developed philosophy and theories of applied psychology. A detailed discussion of these ideas is beyond the scope of this chapter, but in brief they consist of:

- Functional contextualism: the fundamental idea is that all behaviour has a purpose, or function, in context, and focuses on identifying what

purpose a given behaviour serves in each situation. Behaviours are not limited to things that people do, but also include thoughts and emotions.
- Applied behavioural analysis (ABA): ABA is the practical application of functional contextualist ideas; in examining a particular behaviour, the preceding events (antecedents), the behaviour and the consequence are all taken into consideration, along with the context in which the behaviour occurs. These ideas may help people to understand better how their behaviours (both public and private) influence the quality of their lives on a broader scale. By increasing understanding in how these behaviours interact, problematic behaviours can become part of the focus for change.
- Relational frame theory (RFT): a theory of language use which explains how humans relate, or make links between, two or more concepts. In terms of understanding human emotions and behaviour, RFT suggests that humans can have knowledge of things they have never experienced, which can influence their emotions and responses in certain situations.

Drawing on ideas from the above, ACT is based on the central idea that suffering is a normal part of the human experience and is driven by thought and language (Strosahl et al., 2012).

Within ACT, people experiencing emotional distress or displaying problematic behaviours are viewed as responding to the difficult thoughts and feelings that go along with life's challenges in unhelpful and inflexible ways (Harris, 2019). The processes of the human mind that can lead to this are:

- Cognitive fusion: difficulty separating from thoughts and basing responses to situations as if the content of thoughts were real
- Experiential avoidance: attempts to get rid of or away from any internal events, such as thoughts, feelings or memories that are experienced as unpleasant, uncomfortable and unwanted.

ACT emphasises that people can change the way they respond to internal experiences, even in the most difficult of circumstances. In keeping with this, ACT focuses on the present and future, rather than on trying to change things which cannot "unhappen". Psychological flexibility is a central process in ACT and refers to the ability to connect with the present moment in order to engage with value-directed behaviour (Hayes et al., 2012). ACT does not aim to change unpleasant thoughts or feelings; rather, the aim of therapy is often to become more aware of how our reactions to thoughts and feelings can sometimes interfere with living a value-based life. In many cases, the thoughts and feelings themselves may change as a by-product of noticing such experiences, observing them and acknowledging their presence.

The development of psychological flexibility using ACT can be through learning and practising the following range of skills.

Openness

- Acceptance: the ability to observe and pay attention to private events (i.e. thoughts/emotions) without attempting to suppress or change them
- Defusion: identifying inner experiences and thoughts as simply thoughts, rather than the truth; the opposite of cognitive fusion.

Awareness

- Contact with the present moment: shifting attention to the here and now – both internal and external events. Observing these events and understanding that both internal and external experiences are ever-changing
- Self-as-context: the concept that we are more than just our thoughts, emotions, values, judgements and memories. Rather, we are the person who notices and observes such things about ourselves.

Engagement

- Values: clarifying important aspects of life for a person, to help guide and motivate future action
- Committed action: the process of taking concrete steps toward goals, guided by values, despite the potential for unpleasant experiences, for example, anxiety.

In terms of therapeutic work, ACT lends itself to flexible delivery and can be adapted to the needs of the individual and service context. Interventions can be:

- Part of longer-term therapy, either standalone or within an overarching framework, for example, neuropsychological rehabilitation
- Brief pieces of work, drawing on the key processes within ACT, such as identifying and moving toward values, or using a functional contextual approach to determine the function of unwanted behaviours occurring
- Standalone techniques or strategies which aim to develop psychological flexibility.

ACT as a treatment approach for people who have experienced ABI

The experience of physical illness or a long-term health condition such as ABI is often an unwanted, sudden and challenging life event that can impact upon all areas of an individual's life. Understandably, it can be difficult to come to terms with subsequent changes in ability that can impact many domains of functioning and relationships. The primary aim of neuropsychological rehabilitation is to help people navigate and adjust to these difficulties using the skills available to them.

The evidence from research does not conclusively point towards the use of any specific psychological therapy or approach in working with people who have experienced ABI. However, there is a growing body of research that suggests that ACT is useful for people adjusting to long-term physical health conditions (Hann & McCracken, 2014), and ABI specifically (Sander et al., 2020; Whiting et al., 2019).

Both ACT and neuropsychological rehabilitation have strong foundations in behavioural psychology and therefore have similar ways of understanding people and their responses to challenges. In addition, the ideas of functional contextualism reflect the views of Luria, one of the early founders of neuropsychological rehabilitation, who argued that it was important to view the individual and their actions within their social context (see Wilson, 2017). Indeed, Kangas and McDonald (2011) highlight that many of the underlying principles in ACT are consistent with the established principles of neuropsychological rehabilitation.

The range of behavioural and emotional difficulties that are experienced as a result of a brain injury is broad. It can often be difficult to determine which changes are due to the injury itself, and which are due to changes in a person's life as a result of the brain injury, for example change in social life or employment. Whilst many people display a remarkable ability to adapt to changing life situations, some people who have experienced an ABI, just as with some people in the general population, may need a little more support in adjusting. A key focus of rehabilitation is to get people back to previously enjoyed roles and activities, though often changes to physical, emotional or cognitive functioning resulting from the injury may limit the availability of some activities. This change, often experienced as a loss, can understandably be very difficult for people to navigate. Exploring a person's values using ACT can help them to consider why such activities are important to them and to identify alternative activities which are accessible following ABI. As such, this may support the person to feel connected to their values and live their life in a way which is consistent with what is important to them.

Taking a functional contextual approach to understanding behaviour can be experienced as validating for the individual because it considers behaviours within their context and takes a non-blaming stance (Gordon & Borushok, 2017). Incorporating ABA into formulations can be useful in developing an understanding of responses that can be perceived as difficult, to aid in making sense of this for the individual, their family and the services that support them.

It can sometimes be difficult for people to think about new challenges which they face as a result of their brain injury, and to set realistic goals for the future. Understandably, the focus of attention can often be on what used to be for that person, which may give rise to thoughts and feelings that could be considered unpleasant, such as grief or anger about the ABI, and/or a perceived loss of sense of self. The stories that people hold about themselves can often be rigid and inflexible, drawing specific identities and associated roles, actions and ways of being. When faced with a life-changing injury, rigid ideas about the self can make it difficult to adjust to the change in circumstances and live a life based on values. Adjustment to life after a brain injury has been described as accepting new difficulties, adapting behaviour and re-engaging with valued relationships (Antonak et al., 1993), which Whiting et al. (2017) liken to two aspects of psychological flexibility – acceptance and self as context. Practising viewing events from different perspectives may thus be helpful in working with difficulties arising from an attachment to their pre-injury sense of self following ABI. This may also help people to recentre their sense of self according to their values, rather than through specific behaviours (Kangas & McDonald, 2011). Higher levels of acceptance have been associated with a greater quality of life following brain injury (van Bost et al., 2005).

Conclusion

ACT and neuropsychological rehabilitation have both been developed from similar philosophical and scientific underpinnings. They also have in common the overall aim of helping people to live the best possible life despite the difficult situations they find themselves in. From a brain injury context, ACT can promote a focus on living a valued life despite the impact of the brain injury itself, and the challenges and difficulties which life may continue to bring. The integration of ACT within a holistic neuropsychological rehabilitation approach can thus promote values-based cognitive and physical rehabilitation, alongside emotional well-being.

Suggested further reading

Bennett, R., & Oliver, J. E. (2019). *Acceptance and commitment therapy: 100 key points and techniques*. Routledge.

Newby, G., Coetzer, R., Daisley, A., & Weatherhead, S. (2013). *Practical neuropsychological rehabilitation in acquired brain injury: A guide for working clinicians*. Karnac Books.

Wilson, B. A., Winegardner, J., Van Heugten, C. M., & Ownsworth, T. (2017). *Neuropsychological rehabilitation: The international handbook*. Routledge.

References

Antonak, R. F., Livneh, H., & Antonak, C. (1993). A review of research on psychosocial adjustment to impairment in persons with traumatic brain injury. *The Journal of Head Trauma Rehabilitation, 8*(4), 87–100. https://doi.org/10.1097/00001199-199312000-00009

Dindo, L., Van Liew, J. R., & Arch, J. J. (2017). Acceptance and commitment therapy: A transdiagnostic behavioral intervention for mental health and medical conditions. *Neurotherapeutics*, *14*(3), 546–553. https://doi.org/10.1007/s13311-017-0521-3

Freeman, A., Adams, M., & Ashworth, F. (2015). An exploration of the experience of self in the social world for men following traumatic brain injury. *Neuropsychological Rehabilitation*, *25*(2), 189–215. https://doi.org/10.1080/09602011.2014.917686

Gordon, T., & Borushok, J. (2017). *The ACT approach: A comprehensive guide for acceptance and commitment therapy*. PESI Publishing & Media.

Hann, K. E., & McCracken, L. M. (2014). A systematic review of randomized controlled trials of acceptance and commitment therapy for adults with chronic pain: Outcome domains, design quality, and efficacy. *Journal of Contextual Behavioral Science*, *3*(4), 217–227. https://doi.org/10.1016/j.jcbs.2014.10.001

Harris, R. (2019). *ACT made simple: An easy-to-read primer on acceptance and commitment therapy* (2nd ed.). New Harbinger.

Hayes, S. C. (2019). *A liberated mind: How to pivot toward what matters*. Avery.

Hayes, S. C., Luoma, J. B., Bond, F. W., Masuda, A., & Lillis, J. (2006). Acceptance and commitment therapy: Model, processes and outcomes. *Behaviour Research and Therapy*, *44*(1), 1–25. https://doi.org/10.1016/j.brat.2005.06.006

Hayes, S. C., Strosahl, K. D., & Wilson, K. G. (2012). *Acceptance and commitment therapy: The process and practice of mindful change*. Guilford Press.

Headway. (2019). *Acquired brain injury 2016–2017 statistics based on UK admissions*. www.headway.org.uk/about-brain-injury/further-information/statistics/

Jackson, H. F., & Hague, G. (2013). Social consequences and social solutions: Community neuro-rehabilitation in real social environments. In G. Newby, R. Coetzer, A. Daisley, & S. Weatherhead (Eds), *Practical neuropsychological rehabilitation in acquired brain injury: A guide for working clinicians* (pp. 115–156). Routledge.

Kangas, M., & McDonald, S. (2011). Is it time to act? The potential of acceptance and commitment therapy for psychological problems following acquired brain injury. *Neuropsychological Rehabilitation*, *21*(2), 250–276. https://doi.org/10.1080/09602011.2010.540920

National Institute for Health and Care Excellence (NICE). (2014). *Head injury*. Quality standard QS74. www.nice.org.uk/guidance/qs74

Royal College of Physicians & British Society of Rehabilitation Medicine. (2003). *Rehabilitation following acquired brain injury: National clinical guidelines*. https://shop.rcplondon.ac.uk/products/rehabilitation-following-acquired-brain-injury-national-clinical-guidelines?variant=6637228869

Sander, A. M., Clark, A. N., Arciniegas, D. B., Tran, K., Leon-Novelo, L., Ngan, E., Bogaards, J., Sherer, M., & Walser, R. (2020). A randomized controlled trial of acceptance and commitment therapy for psychological distress among persons with traumatic brain injury. *Neuropsychological Rehabilitation*, 1–25. https://doi.org/10.1080/09602011.2020.1762670

Strosahl, K. D., Robinson, P. J., & Gustavsson, T. (2012). *Brief interventions for radical change: Principles and practice of focused acceptance and commitment therapy*. New Harbinger.

van Bost, G., Lorent, G., & Crombez, G. (2005). Aanvaarding na niet-aangeboren hersenletsel. *Gedragstherapie*, *38*(4), 245.

Weatherhead, S., Coezter, R., Daisley, A., Newby, G., Yates, G., & Calvert, P. (2013). Therapy and engagement. In G. Newby, R. Coetzer, A. Daisley, & S. Weatherhead

(Eds.), *Practical neuropsychological rehabilitation in acquired brain injury: A guide for working clinicians* (p. 115). Routledge.

Whiting, D. L., Deane, F. P., McLeod, H. J., Ciarrochi, J., & Simpson, G. K. (2019). Can acceptance and commitment therapy facilitate psychological adjustment after a severe traumatic brain injury? A pilot randomized controlled trial. *Neuropsychological Rehabilitation, 30*(7), 1–24.

Whiting, D. L., Deane, F. P., Simpson, G. K., McLeod, H. J., & Ciarrochi, J. (2017). Cognitive and psychological flexibility after a traumatic brain injury and the implications for treatment in acceptance-based therapies: A conceptual review. *Neuropsychological Rehabilitation, 27*(2), 263–299. https://doi.org/10.1080/09602011.2015.1062115

Wilson, B. A. (2017). The development of neuropsychological rehabilitation. In B. A. Wilson, J. Winegardner, C. M. Van Heugten, & T. Ownsworth (Eds.), *Neuropsychological rehabilitation: The international handbook*. Routledge.

Chapter 3

The Y-Shaped model of psychological adaptation after brain injury

An acceptance and commitment perspective

Fergus Gracey, Katrina Vicentijevic and Abigail Methley

Abstract

Nearly 15 years after its development, the Y-Shaped model remains influential in the integration of identity and emotional changes into neurorehabilitation. Since its inception there has been a growth in "third-wave" psychological therapies such as acceptance and commitment therapy (ACT), applied to the challenges of life post brain injury. In this chapter we outline key principles of the Y-Shaped model alongside those of ACT and illustrate a number of areas of conceptual and technical convergence. A range of ACT-based approaches can be readily integrated into rehabilitation in a way which is informed by the Y-Shaped model, providing coherence to rehabilitation programmes organised around an understanding of human needs and emotions.

The Y-Shaped model was initially proposed as a way to formalise and structure the integration of psychological change into the interdisciplinary rehabilitation process within the Oliver Zangwill Centre holistic rehabilitation programme (Wilson et al., 2009). We hoped the model would also inform choice of process and outcome measurement in rehabilitation more widely and provide a theoretical basis for future research in the area. The original paper (Gracey et al., 2009), has been cited over 140 times (peak year 2019), indicating that it still appears relevant and applicable. It has been cited in reference to a range of intervention models, including third-wave therapeutic approaches to neurological conditions (Robinson et al., 2019), compassion-focused therapy (Ashworth et al., 2011) and valued living (Pais et al., 2019). It provides a tool for collaborative formulation with the rehabilitation team, service users and family members, and materials to facilitate this are now available (Gracey et al., 2017). The model is accessible and applicable to a diverse audience and range of contexts, in part due to the focus on common processes as evidenced in research and clinical practice, rather than conceptualisation based on a single therapeutic model.

DOI: 10.4324/9781003024408-4

Key aspects of the Y-Shaped model

The Y-Shaped model was developed in response to practical challenges to enhancing interdisciplinary working, service user needs (many having some version of "I want the old me back" as a goal), and to integrate contemporary research on emotional outcomes with relevant rehabilitation theory. Goldstein's (1952) holistic theory applied to brain injury described the emotional response to the threat of post-injury changes as a "catastrophic reaction". To protect identity after brain injury, a natural tendency is to avoid triggers, even avoiding "deliberation" or thoughts about the injury. This avoidance can in turn contribute to post-injury disability. With a growing body of evidence that subjective discrepancy (between current and pre-injury or ideal self) and avoidant coping are associated with negative emotional outcomes, we brought together the idea that subjective discrepancy, the existential threat of this and the related understandable behavioural and emotional reactions lie at the heart of many of the frustrations, distress and longer-term restricted outcomes experienced by people with brain injury. The Y-Shaped model outlines a rehabilitation process based on this understanding for integrating rehabilitation activities with emotional adaptation.

The first step in rehabilitation informed by the Y-Shaped model (Gracey et al., 2009) is to understand and address the existential "threat" through therapeutic safety: developing a shared understanding with the person, exploring their experience in different ways and creating the potential to talk about and reflect on their experience rather than simply react. Following a brain injury, some people can reflect on the discrepancy and the distress it causes. Others may avoid or suppress it, or struggle to report their experience due to cognitive and communication changes. This might require careful integration of therapeutic work with cognitive rehabilitation addressing awareness, communication and family work. Once this therapeutic groundwork is done, there is potential for further reduction of the experienced discrepancy through a combination of reduced threat reaction and altered appraisals of what "self after brain injury" and "pre-injury / ideal / aspired-to self" represent. In our experience, the work of reducing avoidance or struggle typically involves some degree of increase in distress "in the moment" whilst the person engages with their hitherto avoided experience, and risk assessment around this might be necessary.

There follows a point where the person reports feeling "the old self has come back" in some partial but recognisable way, representing subjective "resolution" of discrepancy coupled with reduction of the threat reaction to the discrepancy. Following this, the tail of the "Y" highlights rehabilitative efforts that focus on further investment in new or yet-to-be discovered aspects of self that are also connected to "the old self". This can be achieved through a focus on creating the conditions to support participation in activities and relationships, reflection on how these experiences feel and what they mean, and pursuit of further activities that deepen and enrich what is being discovered and learned.

Relational frame theory and its application to post-injury adjustment

The underpinning conceptual basis for acceptance and commitment therapy (ACT) is relational frame theory (RFT; Hayes et al., 2001; Törneke, 2010). RFT is a modern behaviour analytical approach which explains how language influences behaviour, and how language helps us understand relationships between things we have not directly experienced. It is a basic ability of humans to *relate* things, automatically at times, without knowing we are doing it – and as part of this, to relate language to objects or experiences. The relational frame is the expression of the relationship between things. This automatic relating process facilitates our understanding of the world. Once learnt, networks cannot be forgotten and are difficult to inhibit. This can be problematic where we are unable to take a step back from a network to see how it might be unhelpful. Where the relational frame includes emotions such as shame, or negative perceptions of the self as trapped, broken, unlovable, weak or bad, experiences such as anxiety and depression might arise (Hayes & Smith, 2005).

Various ways of relating are described capturing different logical relationships including linking, distinguishing, hierarchical relations and those that depend on context or deictic relations. A particular stimulus can therefore lead to a relational network developing over time which maintains our propensity to respond in a particular way and which therefore might become a focus for therapeutic work. Therefore, within ACT, it is essential to understand the function of any particular stimulus, be that internal or external, in order to provide a helpful intervention. Once the relational frame and stimulus function are understood, it becomes easier to become a "curious observer" of our experiences (including emotions, thoughts, memories and sensations) and the stories we tell about ourselves. A commonly used example is that we are the sky, whilst our experiences are the weather – the weather can change frequently from beautiful sunshine to thunderous storms, but the sky remains a constant throughout.

This conceptual approach can be readily applied to making sense of research regarding relationships of distress to experience of self-discrepancy following brain injury (e.g. Cantor et al., 2005) and how this is related to specific social and activity contexts (Gracey et al., 2008). For example, someone's experience of sadness or frustration triggered by altered abilities in a specific situation could be framed in terms of distinction against "how I used to do this" and might be further elaborated in a relational network to do with loss of worth and pointlessness (e.g. downward social comparison of self to others). Such unpleasant and troubling experiences would be avoided or battled with (through attempts to strive, for example) as a natural human response. Over time, this relational network becomes further elaborated and applied to the association of a particular stimulus (e.g. trying to cook, using a strategy, parenting a young child, talking about return to work) with a particular response (e.g. grief, sadness, frustration, worry). In this way, RFT provides a conceptual basis for formulating identity-related challenges in life post brain injury.

This convergence between the processes outlined in the Y-Shaped model and core intervention principles of ACT is illustrated in Figure 3.1, and a more detailed translation of intervention components is presented in Table 3.1. To further demonstrate application of ACT-based approaches within the Y-Shaped model, a clinical case illustration is now presented.

Clinical illustration

Maja,[1] aged 64 years, suffered a traumatic brain injury (TBI) due to a fall. A CT scan showed a right traumatic subdural haemorrhage, right frontoparietal bore and midline shift. As a consequence of the TBI, she experienced mild dysphonia (changes to her voice), left-sided weakness, limited functional use of her left upper limb and significant pain in her left shoulder. Cognitive changes included difficulties with sustained attention and increased distractibility, an inattention to the left-hand side of her body and cognitive fatigue. These attentional difficulties affected other cognitive domains, such as memory, and would often reduce her capacity to self-monitor in the moment. She also reported anxiety, depression and sense of lost identity.

Maja began a community-based multidisciplinary neurorehabilitation programme 6 months post-injury. When asked about her pre-injury identity, she said her role had always been about caring for others – her husband, daughters, father and friends; and she described herself as the "life and soul of the party". On starting rehabilitation, she described her current self as a "burden", felt she had lost her independence, was struggling to do her usual activities of daily living due to her physical difficulties and was no longer socialising or pursuing her passion of singing. There was a strong sense of feeling "stuck", which resonated with the rehabilitation team who also felt "stuck" about lack of progress in rehabilitation. Psychological therapy sessions, alongside other multidisciplinary team sessions, drew on the Y-Shaped model and ACT principles in considering the presenting issues in terms of identity changes and providing a context in which these could be addressed.

Consistent with the Y-Shaped model, work focused on specific personally important areas. The dysphonia was particularly significant for Maja as she previously sang regularly, and this was a big part of her identity. In order to try to maintain continuity of identity Maja avoided singing altogether, saying

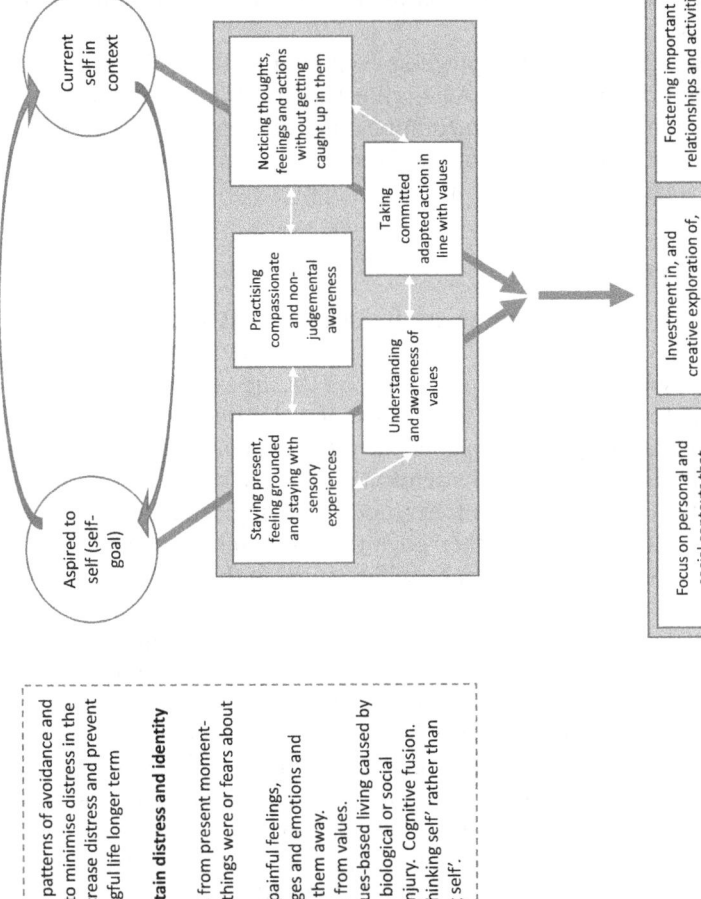

Problem: Stuck in patterns of avoidance and struggle that aim to minimise distress in the short term but increase distress and prevent a rich and meaningful life longer term

Factors that maintain distress and identity discrepancy:
1. Disconnection from present moment-focus on how things were or fears about the future.
2. Struggle with painful feelings, sensations, urges and emotions and trying to push them away.
3. Disconnection from values.
4. Barriers to values-based living caused by psychological, biological or social barriers post injury. Cognitive fusion.
5. Stuck in the 'thinking self' rather than the 'observing self'.

Figure 3.1 An updated version of the Y-Shaped model incorporating acceptance and commitment therapy processes (Gracey et al., 2009; Hayes & Smith, 2005).

Table 3.1 Post-injury challenges, processes of the Y-Shaped model and acceptance and commitment therapy (ACT) principles

Current experience / presenting issue	Target processes for intervention in Y-Shaped model	Related ACT principle
Sense of threat (feared and actual catastrophic meanings of post-injury situation)	Creating therapeutic safety through understanding and compassion	Grounding strategies, self-compassion and staying within the present moment to take a step back from worries and fears
Subjective discrepancy (past/future vs. now)	Reflection on present-moment experiences. Exploration of multiple identities in past, present and potentially future	Focus on present moment; explore other self-narratives; cognitive defusion (disrupting the rigid "frame" in which present and pre-injury selves are unfavourably compared)
Avoidance of thoughts, feelings, sensations, situations which are distressing	Approaching these distressing experiences without avoidance, generating a context for exploration, experimentation and creativity so it feels "safe to explore"	Letting go of the struggle with avoidance (often requiring skills in experiential acceptance) to reflect on the situation and how to take steps towards valued goals despite discomfort
Struggling with distress, clinging to attempts to reduce threat / maintain continuity	Reflecting on understandable coping efforts; exploring conflicts in goals or aspirations generated by these understandable attempts to reduce threat/ maintain continuity; exploring the pros and cons of different attempts to cope	Letting go of any preconceptions about how they "should"respond to challenges and instead non-judgementally asking what they need to do now to live a meaningful and full life. Using creative helplessness. Exploring the risks and benefits of dropping the struggle (often imagined like the rope in a game of tug of war)
Compelled to act (unhelpfully) with limited self-reflection	Able to pause, stop and think, mentally review, potentially scaffolded through rehabilitation strategies or activities embedded in behavioural experiments. Use additional strategies for executive functioning, attention and self-awareness as necessary	Develop mindfulness / metacognitive skills (taking a step back from thoughts and feelings, observing their changeable nature). Use of the choice point diagram to reflect on choices, including understanding any "hooks" that may pull them back

(continued)

Table 3.1 Cont.

Current experience / presenting issue	Target processes for intervention in Y-Shaped model	Related ACT principle
Need for certainty	Ability to tolerate uncertainty, use of "experimentation", play, exploration. Fostering curiosity about the unknown	Developing skills in mindfulness, committed and values-based action even when the outcome is uncertain, and developing psychological flexibility
Rigid hope for the "old self", and feelings of loss or grief	Capacity to open up possibility of "new self"; experiments in rehabilitation / therapy to explore this experientially. Respond to understandable emotions that arise	Acceptance of emotional experience and opening up to the possibility of developing a "new self" despite the pain and loss experienced
Disconnection from sense of identity	Reconnection to identities through experiences that indicate new or different possibilities for enacting important aspects of identities. Identifying situations that nourish specific identities	Developing a clear awareness of pre-injury values and how these can be met (often through adapted activity) post brain injury. Focus on activities as source of "self" and motivating values enables a positive identity despite these changes
Avoidance of opportunities, resulting in lack of positive meanings and emotions and further detachment from everyday life	Developing a blueprint to further explore identity work (as above) in life post-rehabilitation. Use of memory strategies to support reflection on, and engagement with, new experiences	Taking committed action towards valued goals, despite the discomfort caused. Increased opportunity to develop meaning, experience positive emotions and interactions and develop a new sense of identity

she wanted to "wait" until her voice got better. The description of "waiting" also provided a safe way of understanding the relationship between the brain injury and not singing, reducing immediate threat to identity. However, the avoidance and "framing" of the loss of singing in this way reduced her engagement in meaningful activity, and progress with rehabilitation (e.g. avoiding the exercises needed to strengthen her vocal muscles). This led to a further sense of disconnection from this core part of her sense of identity, as well as increased self-critical thoughts and worry about getting better. This pattern was also observed in other personally important areas and helped explain getting "stuck" in rehabilitation progress due to various forms of avoidance or unhelpful framing.

Through reflection on this formulation, Maja was able to understand how investing all her efforts into reducing feelings of discrepancy took her further away from the meaningful activity she wanted. Psychological intervention focused on skills in witnessing thoughts, feelings and actions without getting "hooked", stepping back or "defusion" from critical thoughts, mindfulness, acceptance of distressing experiences whilst reducing avoidance, and promoting committed action towards personally valued activities. Part of this work involved Maja exploring singing in "safe" circumstances, such as singing meaningful songs on her own at home. By observing and accepting how that felt, she began to visualise what performing to an audience again might look and feel like. Creatively exploring this possible future identity seemed to allow her to take further steps towards this values-based goal.

Maja changed the way she saw herself and her relationship with her thoughts and feelings, opening up to the possibility of developing a "new self" despite the pain and loss experienced. As such her "framing" of her post-injury self shifted from one of negative comparison and distinction from pre-injury. This helped her to be more accepting on the "bad" days when she was experiencing threat to her identity or grieving for losses. Maja was also able to begin to re-engage with singing in an adapted way and became more accepting of her "new voice", gaining positive meanings and interactions. At the point of discharge, Maja's mood was improving, and she seemed to be nourishing a new sense of identity as a singer and performer, as well as beginning to re-engage socially and provide some care to others in her life.

Conclusion

In our discussions of the Y-Shaped model and its application we have considered some key points of convergence with developments in the application of ACT in neurorehabilitation. In this chapter we have set out components of the Y-Shaped model mapped on to an ACT-based understanding of adaptation to life post-injury. In so doing we feel we have both enhanced the descriptive power of the Y-Shaped model and signposted readers to a wider range of techniques that could be applied in creating contexts which ultimately support people to lead lives that are fulfilling and rewarding despite the inevitable restrictions of their brain injury.

Note

1 Some real-world clinical examples have been used to illustrate the points raised in this chapter; names and identifying details have been changed and/or amalgamated with other examples to protect confidentiality.

Suggested further reading

Goldstein, K. (1952). The effects of brain damage on the personality. *Psychiatry: Journal for the Study of the Interpersonal Processes, 15*(3), 245–260. https://doi.org/10.1080/00332747.1952.11022878

Owen, R. (2014). *Living with the enemy.* Routledge. https://doi.org/10.4324/9780203797976

Wilson, B. A., Gracey, F., Evans, J. J., & Bateman, A. (2009). *Neuropsychological rehabilitation: Theory, models, therapy and outcome.* Cambridge University Press. https://doi.org/10.1017/CBO9780511581083

References

Ashworth, F., Gracey, F., & Gilbert, P. (2011). Compassion focused therapy after traumatic brain injury: Theoretical foundations and a case illustration. *Brain Impairment, 12*(2), 128–139. https://doi.org/10.1375/brim.12.2.128

Cantor, J. B., Ashman, T. A., Schwartz, M. E., Gordon, W. A., Hibbard, M. R., Brown, M., & Cheng, Z. (2005). The role of self-discrepancy theory in understanding post-traumatic brain injury affective disorders: A pilot study. *The Journal of Head Trauma Rehabilitation, 20*(6), 527–543. https://doi.org/10.1097/00001199-200511000-00005

Goldstein, K. (1952). The effects of brain damage on the personality. *Psychiatry: Journal for the Study of the Interpersonal Processes, 15*(3), 245–260. https://doi.org/10.1080/00332747.1952.11022878

Gracey, F., Evans, J. J., & Malley, D. (2009). Capturing processes and outcome in complex rehabilitation interventions: A "Y-shaped model". *Neuropsychological Rehabilitation, 19*(6), 867–890. https://doi.org/10.1080/09602010903027763

Gracey, F., Palmer, S., Rous, B., Psaila, K., Shaw, K., O'Dell, J., & Mohamed, S. (2008). "Feeling part of things": Personal construction of self after brain injury. Neuropsychological Rehabilitation, 18(5–6), 627–650. https://doi.org/10.1080/09602010903027763

Gracey, F., Prince, L., & Winson, R. (2017). Working with identity change after brain injury. In R. Winson, B. A. Wilson, & A. Bateman (Eds.), *The brain injury rehabilitation workbook* (p. 282). Guilford. https://doi.org/10.4324/9781315172897

Hayes, S. C., Barnes-Holmes, D., & Roche, B. (2001). *Relational frame theory: A post-Skinnerian account of human language and cognition.* Kluwer Academic/Plenum. https://doi.org/10.1007/b108413

Hayes, S., & Smith, S. (2005). *Get out of your mind and into your life: The new acceptance and commitment therapy.* New Harbinger. https://doi.org/10.1016/s1155-1704(07)89715-1

Pais, C., Ponsford, J. L., Gould, K. R., & Wong, D. (2019). Role of valued living and associations with functional outcome following traumatic brain injury. *Neuropsychological Rehabilitation, 29*(4), 625–637. https://doi.org/10.1080/09602011.2017.1313745

Robinson, P., Russell, A., & Dysch, L. (2019). Third-wave therapies for long-term neurological conditions: A systematic review to evaluate the status and quality of evidence. *Brain Impairment, 20*(1), 58–80. https://doi.org/10.1017/brimp.2019.2

Törneke, N. (2010). *Learning RFT: An introduction to relational frame theory and its clinical application.* Context Press. https://doi.org/10.1016/j.cbpra.2011.05.004

Wilson, B. A., Gracey, F., Malley, D., Bateman, A., & Evans, J. J. (2009). The Oliver Zangwill Centre approach to neuropsychological rehabilitation. In B. Wilson, F. Gracey, J. J. Evans, & A. Bateman (Eds.), *Neuropsychological rehabilitation: Theory, models, therapy and outcome.* Cambridge University Press. https://doi.org/10.1017/cbo9780511581083.003

Part II

Adapting ACT approaches for neuropsychological presentations

Acceptance and commitment therapy with children who have experienced brain injury

Victoria Gray and Ingram Wright

Abstract

This chapter will offer insights into the ways acceptance and commitment therapy (ACT) might be adapted for use with children with brain injury across a range of developmental stages, including considerations for how ACT might support assessment, rehabilitation and emotional wellbeing. The use of ACT within child brain injury rehabilitation brings exciting opportunities to explore creative ways to support young people who have experienced a life-changing event.

Acquired brain injuries (ABIs) in childhood have an incidence of 82 per 100,000 children per year, with 18 of these being of traumatic origin. Approximately 500 children and young people are diagnosed with a brain tumour each year in the UK (Stiller et al., 2019). Epilepsy, the common significant long-term neurological condition of childhood, affects 1 in 220 children or approximately 55,000 children and young people in the UK (Meeraus et al., 2013).

Due to treatment advances, survival rates for all forms of childhood ABI are improving dramatically. For example, survival following treatment for a childhood brain tumour is now over 72% (Ostrom et al., 2015). However, such survival is associated with significant cognitive and emotional difficulties. Large numbers of children and young people live with learning and behavioural problems alongside cognitive impairments such as attentional problems, visuospatial processing difficulties and memory deficits. Physical symptoms such as fatigue, motor control problems and communication difficulties are commonly coupled with psychological problems such as anxiety, depression and post-traumatic stress (Bruce et al., 2011; Turner et al., 2009).

Emotional and mental health problems are highly prevalent in children with any chronic health condition and such difficulties are specifically amplified in any conditions with neurological components (Wright, 2018). Many childhood ABIs are associated with significant cognitive problems, acquired

DOI: 10.4324/9781003024408-6

learning disabilities and corresponding poor educational progress. Co-occurring neurodevelopmental problems such as attention deficit disorder, social communication disorders and autism are common. Anxiety and mood disturbance is often identified from early in adolescence and into adulthood (Leclezio et al., 2015; Luis & Mittenberg, 2002).

At the psychosocial level, there is increasing evidence of the impact of paediatric ABI on social and educational functioning, self-esteem, parental stress and broader family functioning. Difficulties experienced by children injured in their early years are often amplified in adolescence due to a combination of maturational challenges in brain development and increasing environmental expectations, in terms of social, cognitive and emotional functioning at home and at school. For example, communication difficulties and associated impairments in social functioning can contribute to social anxiety and consequent isolation (Bonner et al., 2008; Gurney et al., 2009; Schulte & Barrera, 2010). The combined impact of these effects has led children with ABI to have higher rates of educational failure, lower levels of adult independence and amongst the poorest health-related quality of life in adulthood (Anderson et al., 2011; Klonoff et al., 1993).

Despite the high prevalence of psychological and psychosocial problems following ABI, access to mental health services for children with physical health conditions and acquired brain injury is heavily constrained (Garralda, 2004). In neurological conditions, the relationship between an underlying condition and the presenting mental health or emotional problems is often poorly understood. As a consequence, children's difficulties are either not recognised or the presence of an ABI leads to exclusion from mental health services. These kinds of restrictions are not so much based on scarce resources but intrinsic preconceptions in service delivery that interventions must respect the relationship between an underlying mental health problem and the underlying aetiology of the neurological condition. It is often assumed that treatments appropriate for children with primary mental health problems may be ineffective in children with co-existing health or neurological conditions. Additional barriers include geographical challenges to access specialist support which recognises the complexity of the interaction.

A broad range of post-injury problems are experienced by children following ABI, which may be lifelong. There is a clear need for evidence of efficacious treatments to support young people through the developmentally important transition from childhood to adulthood. Although there are evident barriers to healthcare access, there is a small but increasing evidence for efficacy of psychological interventions which are specifically designed to meet the needs of children with neurological conditions (Dorris et al., 2017; Fonagy & Clark, 2015).

The application of ACT principles to paediatric brain injury

Acceptance and commitment therapy (ACT) has a growing evidence base for its efficacy in the treatment of children and adolescents with health conditions, In many cases, ACT had proved to have longer-term benefits superior to cognitive-behavioural therapy (CBT) which is potentially constrained in its application to children with health conditions (Swain et al., 2015).

ACT is an evidence-based psychological therapy that has been successfully used to improve physical and mental health among children and adults with chronic conditions, including brain injuries (Bond et al., 2006; Coyne et al., 2011; Feros et al., 2013; Graham et al., 2016; Hulbert-Williams et al., 2015). ACT is a "third-wave" CBT that encourages openness to and awareness of the present moment in order to help participants maintain behaviours consistent with their life goals (Hayes et al., 2016). ACT fosters engagement with, rather than avoidance of, painful experiences to move towards acceptance of unchangeable difficulties alongside building a rich and meaningful life despite the presence of ongoing difficulties (Bond et al., 2006). This gives ACT strong face validity for application for people with ABI, where there can be permanent cognitive difficulties and unavoidable physical and functional impairments.

In paediatric services, ACT has been used to support young people with a wide range of long-term symptoms of chronic disease (Swain et al., 2015). Use of such third-wave approaches with young people is well established (e.g. Epston et al., 1997). Models grounded in contextual behavioural science principles have also been developed with child and adolescent populations in mind, for example, DNA-V (referring to discovery, noticer, advisor, values; Ciarrochi et al., 2016). The "acceptance" encouraged in ACT is specifically associated with improved post-treatment functioning in young people with ABI (Aerts et al., 2019). Overall, current evidence indicates that ACT is clinically effective and targets key response styles that support improved functioning in children with neurological conditions. However, there is currently very limited specific intervention research using ACT with children with neurological conditions who often experience a unique combination of cognitive and psychological difficulties.

Children and young people with ABI (or other neurological conditions) and their families often describe difficulties accommodating changes in the young person's functioning. Seeing this within an ACT framework, the child or their family can become fixed on unworkable actions or ruminate on what has been lost following injury or illness. They may describe difficulties staying connected with the present moment, being drawn to grieve for the loss of a previously anticipated future and being fearful of a new, uncertain, future. Families and the young person have to live with uncertainty and often report that living in the "now" without being overwhelmed by what was, or fearing what might be, can be extremely challenging. Children and families commonly describe feeling anxious that if they "accept" that physical or cognitive difficulties will not resolve, it will take away hope and prevent them striving to make progress in a rehabilitation journey. Such difficulties can leave the child and their family struggling to engage with their values and to make choices towards committed action.

Grief, sadness, fear and anxiety are emotions that are common in a paediatric brain injury population, for the young person and their family. If the young person and their family become "hooked" by these emotions the young person is less likely to engage with and achieve their rehabilitation potential. They may see themselves without context and become fused with thoughts of "I'm not the same me as before", narrowly defining themselves as "just" a person with a brain injury. Behavioural change and experimental avoidance are also seen in a physical rehabilitation context, as the young person becomes more aware of what they are currently unable to do. Frustration can lead to anger, low mood and a drive to disengage from therapy sessions. Similar presenting difficulties and challenges can be present following diagnosis and treatment of other brain injuries such as a brain tumour, stroke or epilepsy. Clinicians utilising ACT to support therapeutic work in this area can help to reshape an understanding of "acceptance" and support the young person to focus on their underlying values to guide their rehabilitative journey and future goals. This can be useful for the young person directly, but can also help to support the systems around the child, such as their family, the therapy team and school.

When working with children and young people with a brain injury or a neurological condition it is important to adapt delivery of therapeutic sessions to allow for common cognitive or functional difficulties. Language and techniques used will need to be adapted appropriately to the developmental level – from pre-school to older adolescent. If the young person has difficulties with verbal processing, then presenting information in a tactile or visual format or providing visual notes for a session will be of particular value in promoting engagement and understanding. For example, working with cartoons can be helpful when explaining metaphors. Modelling clay or craft materials can help to illustrate abstract ideas in a tangible way, such as making or drawing the leaves from the commonly used cognitive defusion technique of "leaves on the stream" (Harris, 2019). If the child or young person has visual difficulties, then work within a predominantly verbal modality, being mindful to repeat information regularly to enhance encoding and recall or recording audio information in voice notes on a smart phone or tablet. A young person with a brain injury may have significant or subtle difficulties within attention and executive functioning domains. Simple strategies can help ameliorate difficulties, such as providing short breaks, giving notes or photographs of output from activities, taking additional time to deliver information and concepts and shortening length/increasing frequency of appointments.

The ACT concept of "values" may be difficult for some children or young people to grasp initially. Using a values list to open up the conversation can be helpful. Ask lots of "what", "how" and "why" questions. For example, with worries about dropping behind at school you might ask, "what is it about doing well at school that is important to you?", "why do you want to do well?", "what makes you want to keep up at school?", "how do you go about doing well at school?" It may help the young person to draw a visual representation of their values and keep them with them, physically as well as metaphorically, to help with grounding and retention of information. The use of ACT conversation cards, physically or virtually, can also support to both open up discussion and retain salient information.

When appropriate, including the wider family in therapy sessions can assist in generalising benefits from the therapy room to everyday life. It can also indirectly or directly help the parents to develop a framework to understand their child's emotions as well as their own. Many aspects of ACT inherently support therapeutic work with children with neurological conditions, such as availability of video clips to aid explanation, visual material to support verbal explanations and enabling modelling and immersive learning through acting out examples together in sessions. As within other therapeutic approaches (e.g. narrative therapy), there is lots of scope for creativity and innovation, drawing on areas or topics that the young person is interested in or enthusiastic about.

Spending time thinking about and identifying goals should not be underestimated when working with this population. As previously highlighted, goals may be significantly different from pre-injury or may need to be adjusted as skills fail to develop naturally or the gap between the young person and peers becomes wider. The authors have used a range of metaphors to support goal work. For example, a road metaphor was used when working with Lucy,[1] a 10-year-old girl who was in a car accident. This helped create an open dialogue about goals between Lucy and her clinical psychologist, and facilitated connection with different aspects of ACT.

Lucy initially presented with high levels of anxiety and a sense of loss, associated with changes in her cognitive and physical functioning. A road was drawn out with Lucy during session to support therapeutic conversations. The metaphor helped to contain uncertainty by breaking goals down along the road, working on one, without ruling out the possibility of a bigger future goal. This allowed space for discussion about goals that might be "mission impossible" at that time, but enabled her curiosity and hope to remain for the future. It opened conversations about addressing "unworkable strategies" and to think how Lucy could choose a good journey to focus on at that time. Lucy was introduced to the concept of "being present" and supported to be on the road without looking back at different routes or looking too far ahead and worrying what might be around the corner. The road helped to make this abstract concept more tangible.

When talking about thoughts or emotions that may "hook" us and lead us away from our goals, it was helpful to talk about choice points (Harris, 2019). Lucy's choice points were drawn as a roundabout with several roads leading from it. The roundabout helped encourage Lucy to stop and consider the route she was being hooked towards, which helped her to identify and practise strategies to help make "moves towards" her goal. Aspects of impulsivity were addressed to support Lucy to notice and employ strategies when needed. This theme was built on to think about challenges that Lucy may come across on her "road" to her goals, and to introduce the concept of committed action. Challenges were drawn in the form of metaphorical bollards or potholes on the road towards Lucy's goals. Lucy was supported to see how roads that avoided the challenges and took her "away" from her goals may be smoother, but ultimately unhelpful and eventually leading away from her goal.

The concept of values was also introduced metaphorically, by asking Lucy what was the "drive" towards her goal. Conversations about self as context were introduced through thinking about what remained the same about her as a person, regardless of which road she was on or who/what else was on the road at that time. Signs were drawn at the side of the road containing difficult thoughts and emotions. Lucy recognised that if she spent too much time reading or looking at the signs, or spent all her energy trying never to look at them, she stopped noticing where she was going or ran out of power to get to her next destination. Lucy found that her motivation to engage in meaningful educational and daily tasks improved and her anxiety reduced. Lucy identified that she had enjoyed coming to the sessions and reflected that it had felt useful to draw out "her" map – indicating that she felt a sense of ownership and involvement in what had been a collaborative process.

The authors have recognised that when working with a child or young person with ABI it allows you to be creative in the deployment of ACT concepts, though it is important to avoid introducing too many novel concepts too quickly. For example, when working with Michael, a 15-year-old boy with multiple sclerosis, a football theme was used to support the therapeutic process. Loosely based on the "hands" metaphor described by Harris (2019), Michael was asked the following:

Imagine you are holding the football and all these thoughts and emotions are contained in it. Hold it to your face. What do you notice? What else is on the pitch? Where is the goal? Where are your supporters? Now place it down. Notice your teammates. Notice your supporters. Can you see the goal that you are moving towards? Can your teammates and supporters help? What skills can you notice that might help?

The football theme was also used to introduce and discuss the concept of acceptance, by imagining difficult thoughts and emotions as people invading the pitch and running around. Michael identified that these pitch invaders got in the way of the goal, and made it harder for him to see his teammates. He recognised that if he only focused on the pitch invaders, he would be unable to focus on the game and would struggle to get closer to scoring a goal. If all his time and energy were spent chasing the pitch invaders off the pitch, he would be less able to enjoy playing or engaging with his teammates.

When thinking about committed action and values, Michael was directed to think about a hypothetical article in the newspaper about himself. The article was not about the number of goals he scored or tackles he made but about him as a person. Michael was asked questions like:

What would you want it to say? What motivates you as a player? What is important to you when your team play? Why is it important to you to do well or support the team? How do you cope with not winning every match?

Michael was supported to connect with the present moment through focusing on the current moment of the game – focusing not on thinking back to what had happened in a previous match and what had or had not gone well, or thinking ahead to if he won or lost, but bringing his attention on to the ball at his feet in this moment, here and now. Mindfulness and breathing exercises were used to support this work. The football theme allowed for recognition of self as context, through discussions about what "endured" about Michael:

What stays even if you play in a different stadium? Or if you have different players around you on the pitch? Or if you have a manager with different expectations, who asks you to play in a different way?

Michael initially presented with significant low mood and self-harming behaviour. Themes of anger, loss, grief, fear of loss of future and living with uncertainty emerged during the assessment. Michael experienced high levels of pain and fatigue and difficulties with attention, memory, planning and problem solving. The intervention resulted in a significantly lower incidence of self-harming behaviour, improvement in mood and a higher level of participation in meaningful activities.

Working with parents and carers

Involvement of parents in sessions and tasks can enable the family to share experiences, reducing parents' feelings of hopelessness or inability to create change. Mindfulness to support grounding can work well as a family and encourages the child to structure it into their day. ACT approaches can also be used to support the parents of a young person with brain injury or a neurological condition specifically with their own emotional adjustment to what may be an incredibly difficult situation.

It may also be necessary for the majority of the work to take place with the parent or carer, for example if the child is very young or unable to participate in therapy due to extent of the injury. Often these ways of working are integrated together, especially if the parent or carer is more focused on caring for their child at the cost of their own emotional needs.

For example, Jennifer, the parent of Ben, a toddler who experienced a hypoxic brain injury with significant functional impact, talked about the importance of holding on to hope whilst being aware that the developmental trajectory for Ben was going to be very different. Jennifer knew that Ben would require lifelong support with all activities of daily living. Jennifer experienced strong emotions of guilt and grief, alongside fear of acceptance. She struggled to come to the hospital ward to sit in the "now" and to be present with Ben.

Jennifer was provided with a therapeutic space to acknowledge her own sadness and grief, and to explore how she may be fused with thoughts of blame and anger. When these thoughts and emotions became overwhelming she was unable to stay by Ben's bedside. Jennifer described feeling disgust at her behaviour and experienced episodes of low mood as a result. Therapy was used to explore her values and she identified the core values of wanting to "do her best for Ben" and to "give Ben love and care". Jennifer was able to explore how grief and sadness were understandable and normal emotional responses in the situation, and were directly connected to the love she felt for Ben. She talked about how these waves of emotion took over when at Ben's bedside, and reflected on how she wanted to learn to "ride" these waves without being as overwhelmed by them. She reflected on how these thoughts and feelings were hooking her away from being present for Ben and inhibiting her in providing love and care in a tangible way. Jennifer worked on strategies of defusion to support her to drop the struggle and enable her to be "present". She worked on imagining her thoughts and emotions being moved into balloons in the cubicle. This helped her to see her thoughts as things that were not fixed, but allowed to float by or come and go, as they needed to. Recognising that being in a better place herself would mean she was more able to love and care for Ben as she wanted to, Jennifer worked on grounding techniques and increased her ability to notice when to employ them. The intervention supported Jennifer to be present with Ben and to tune into how she was able to show Ben the love, care and affection she knew that he needed.

Conclusion

ACT has clear applications to the challenges faced by young people and their families following ABI. Although many techniques deployed within the ACT framework may require adaptation, ACT can be useful in supporting the young person themselves as well as promoting understanding with their families, multidisciplinary teams and wider systems. Many of the young people and families in the ABI population are incredibly resilient and will bring their own ideas and strengths to therapy. The use of ACT within child brain injury intervention and rehabilitation brings exciting opportunities to explore creative ways to support young people who have experienced a life-changing event.

Note

1 Some real-world clinical examples have been used to illustrate the points raised in this chapter; names and identifying details have been changed and/or amalgamated with other examples to protect confidentiality.

Suggested further reading

Bell, M., & Turrell, S. (2016). *ACT for adolescents: Treating teens and adolescents in individual and group therapy.* New Harbinger.

Epston, D., Freeman, J., & Lobovits, D. (1997). *Playful approaches to serious problems: Narrative therapy with children and their families.* WW Norton.

Hayes, L., & Ciarrochi, J. (2015). *The thriving adolescent.* New Harbinger.

Hobday, A., & Ollier, K. (2000). *Creative therapy: Activities with children and adolescents.* Blackwell.

References

Aerts, H., Van Vrekhem, T., Stas, L., & Marinazzo, D. (2019). The interplay between emotion regulation, emotional well-being, and cognitive functioning in brain tumor patients and their caregivers: An exploratory study. *Psycho-Oncology, 28*(10), 2068–2075. https://doi.org/10.1002/pon.5195

Anderson, V., Brown, S., Newitt, H., & Hoile, H. (2011). Long-term outcome from childhood traumatic brain injury: Intellectual ability, personality and quality of life. *Neuropsychology, 25*(2), 176–184. https://doi.org/10.1037/a0021217

Bond, F. W., Hayes, S. C., & Barnes-Holmes, D. (2006). Psychological flexibility, ACT, and organizational behavior. *Journal of Organizational Behavior Management, 26*, 25–54. https://doi.org/10.1300/j075v26n01_02

Bonner, M. J., Hardy, K. K., Willard, V. W., Anthony, K. K., Hood, M., & Gururangan, S. (2008). Social functioning and facial expression recognition in survivors of pediatric brain tumors. *Journal of Pediatric Psychology, 33*(10), 1142–1152. https://doi.org/10.1093/jpepsy/jsn035

Bruce, M., Gumley, D., Isham, L., Fearon, P., & Phipps, K. (2011). Post-traumatic stress symptoms in childhood brain tumour survivors and their parents. *Child: Care, Health and Development, 37*(2), 244–251. https://doi.org/10.1111/j.1365-2214.2010.01164.x

Ciarrochi, J., Atkins, P., Hayes, L., Sahdra, B., & Parker, P. (2016). Contextual positive psychology: Policy recommendations for implementing positive psychology into schools. *Frontiers in Psychology, 7,* 1561. https://doi.org/10.3389/fpsyg.2016.01561

Coyne, L. W., McHugh, L., & Martinez, E. R. (2011, April). Acceptance and commitment therapy (ACT): Advances and applications with children, adolescents, and families. *Child and Adolescent Psychiatric Clinics of North America, 20*(2), 379–399. https://doi.org/10.1016/j.chc.2011.01.010

Dorris, L., Broome, H., Wilson, M., Grant, C., Young, D., Baker, G., ... Wright, I. (2017). A randomized controlled trial of a manual-based psychosocial group intervention for young people with epilepsy [PIE]. *Epilepsy and Behavior, 72*, 89–98. http://dx.doi.org/10.1016/j.yebeh.2017.04.007

Epston, D., Freeman, J., & Lobovits, D. (1997). *Playful approaches to serious problems: Narrative therapy with children and their families.* W. W. Norton.

Feros, D. L., Lane, L., Ciarrochi, J., & Blackledge, J. T. (2013). Acceptance and commitment therapy (ACT) for improving the lives of cancer patients: A preliminary study. *Psycho-Oncology, 22*(2), 459–464. https://doi.org/10.1002/pon.2083

Fonagy, P., & Clark, D. M. (2015). Update on the Improving Access to Psychological Therapies programme in England: Commentary on ... Children and Young People's Improving Access to Psychological Therapies. *BJPsych Bulletin, 39*(5), 248–251. https://doi.org/10.1192/pb.bp.115.052282

Garralda, M. E. (2004). The interface between physical and mental health problems and medical help seeking in children and adolescents: A research perspective. *Child and Adolescent Mental Health, 9*(4), 146–155. http://doi.wiley.com/10.1111/j.1475-3588.2004.00098.x

Graham, C. D., Gouick, J., Krahé, C., & Gillanders, D. (2016). A systematic review of the use of acceptance and commitment therapy (ACT) in chronic disease and long-term conditions. *Clinical Psychology Review, 46*, 46–58. https://doi.org/10.1016/j.cpr.2016.04.009

Gurney, J. G., Krull, K. R., Kadan-Lottick, N., Nicholson, H. S., Nathan, P. C., Zebrack, B., ... Ness, K. K. (2009). Social outcomes in the childhood cancer survivor study cohort. *Journal of Clinical Oncology, 27*, 2390–2395. https://doi.org/10.1200/jco.2008.21.1458

Harris, R. (2019). *ACT made simple* (2nd ed.). New Harbinger.

Hayes, S. C., Strosahl, K. D., & Wilson, K. G. (2016). *Acceptance and commitment therapy: The process and practice of mindful change* (2nd ed.). Guilford.

Hulbert-Williams, N. J., Storey, L., & Wilson, K. G. (2015). Psychological interventions for patients with cancer: Psychological flexibility and the potential utility of acceptance and commitment therapy. *European Journal of Cancer Care, 24*, 15–27. https://doi.org/10.1111/ecc.12223

Klonoff, H., Clark, C., & Klonoff, P. S. (1993). Long-term outcome of head injuries: A 23 year follow up study of children with head injuries. *Journal of Neurology, Neurosurgery and Psychiatry, 56*(4), 410–415. https://doi.org/10.1136/jnnp.56.4.410

Leclezio, L., Jansen, A., Whittemore, V. H., & De Vries, P. J. (2015). Pilot validation of the tuberous sclerosis-associated neuropsychiatric disorders (TAND) checklist. *Pediatric Neurology, 52*(1), 16–24. https://doi.org/10.1016/j.pediatrneurol.2014.10.006

Luis, C. A., & Mittenberg, W. (2002). Mood and anxiety disorders following pediatric traumatic brain injury: A prospective study. *Journal of Clinical and Experimental Neuropsychology, 24*(3), 270–279. https://doi.org/10.1076/jcen.24.3.270.982

Meeraus, W. H., Petersen, I., Chin, R. F., Knott, F., & Gilbert, R. (2013). Childhood epilepsy recorded in primary care in the UK. *Archives of Disease in Childhood*, *98*(3), 195–202. https://doi.org/10.1136/archdischild-2012-302237

Ostrom, Q. T., Gittleman, H., Fulop, J., Liu, M., Blanda, R., Kromer, C., ... Barnholtz-Sloan, J. S. (2015). CBTRUS statistical report: Primary brain and central nervous system tumors diagnosed in the United States in 2008–2012. *Neuro-Oncology*, *17*(Suppl 4), iv1–iv62. https://doi.org/10.1093/neuonc/nov189

Schulte, F., & Barrera, M. (2010). Social competence in childhood brain tumor survivors: A comprehensive review. *Supportive Care in Cancer*, 18, 1499–1513. https://doi.org/10.1007/s00520-010-0963-1

Stiller, C. A., Bayne, A. M., Chakrabarty, A., Kenny, T., & Chumas, P. (2019). Incidence of childhood CNS tumours in Britain and variation in rates by definition of malignant behaviour: Population-based study. *BMC Cancer*, *19*(1), 139. https://doi.org/10.1186/s12885-019-5344-7

Swain, J., Hancock, K., Dixon, A., & Bowman, J. (2015). Acceptance and commitment therapy for children: A systematic review of intervention studies. *Journal of Contextual Behavioral Science*, 4, 73–85. https://doi.org/10.1016/j.jcbs.2015.02.001

Turner, C. D., Rey-Casserly, C., Liptak, C. C., & Chordas, C. (2009). Late effects of therapy for pediatric brain tumor survivors. *Journal of Child Neurology*, *24*(11), 1455–1463. https://pubmed.ncbi.nlm.nih.gov/19841433/

Wright, I. (2018). Paediatric convulsive status epilepticus, epilepsy, and behavioural outcomes. *Developmental Medicine & Child Neurology*, *60*(4), 338–339. https://doi.org/10.1111/dmcn.13700

Chapter 5

Acceptance and commitment therapy for people with mild traumatic brain injury and post-concussion symptoms

Lorraine King and Lindsay Prescott

Abstract

Persistent post-concussion symptoms (PPCS) are common following mild traumatic brain injury, maintained by a complex interplay of physical and psychological processes. Research evidence for effective treatment remains limited, despite the significant burden such symptoms have on people's well-being. Acceptance and commitment therapy (ACT) appears to be a beneficial therapeutic approach in working with this population, although there is a limited empirical evidence base to date. Practice examples from the authors are offered to illustrate the potential usefulness of ACT when working with individuals experiencing PPCS.

Every year in the UK, approximately 1.4 million people suffer a traumatic brain injury (TBI) with 80% diagnosed as mild in severity (National Institute for Health and Care Excellence [NICE], 2019). Mild traumatic brain injury (mTBI) is classified based on the following characteristics of the injury:

- Altered or brief loss of consciousness, of less than 30 minutes
- Glasgow Coma Scale (GCS; a measure of consciousness, assessing eye, verbal and motor responses; Teasdale & Jennett, 1974) score of 13/15 or above, indicating the person is mostly fully alert and responsive immediately after regaining consciousness (but potentially with mild changes in verbal responses, such as confusion or disorientation)
- A duration of post-traumatic amnesia (PTA; a period of post-TBI confusion and inability to remember new information) of less than 24 hours (see McCrea, 2008).

Many people experience post-concussion symptoms following mTBI. Symptoms span physical, cognitive and emotional domains, typically including headaches, dizziness, sleep disturbance, sensitivity to light and/or noise, irritability, and memory and concentration difficulties. Symptoms usually resolve naturally within several days/weeks; however, for an estimated

DOI: 10.4324/9781003024408-7

10–25% of people (Boake et al., 2005), difficulties continue to become persistent post-concussion symptoms (PPCS; Lannsjo et al., 2009).

Theoretical understandings of PPCS

It has proved difficult to define the difficulties that people can experience following mTBI. Varied (and often contradictory) terminology continues to be used within clinical practice. The term persistent post-concussion symptoms was chosen for this chapter to describe chronic difficulties, which continue beyond the duration which would typically be expected from the neurological consequences of a mild brain injury. PPCS are non-specific and have been shown to overlap with symptom clusters of several non-neurological patient groups, including healthy controls (Dean et al., 2012; Iverson & Lange, 2003), people experiencing chronic pain (Radanov et al., 1992), people experiencing depression (Iverson, 2006) and people making personal injury claims that do not involve TBI (Dunn et al., 1995).

In terms of understanding how PPCS develops, it is important to acknowledge the complex interplay between biological, psychological and social factors (Polinder et al., 2018; Silverberg & Iverson, 2011). Some writers purport a subtle neurological aetiology (Hellstrøm et al., 2017; Reuben et al., 2014), and mTBI may lead to damage which is not visible on a routine computed tomography (CT) or magnetic resonance imaging (MRI) scan. Richter et al. (2021) identified potential neuroanatomical substrates of mTBI in white-matter volume and integrity via MRI and highlighted how this evolved in the 2–3 weeks following injury. This study identified that these changes were most closely associated with clinical recovery if MRI scans were performed within 72 hours, yet this early imaging is rarely offered following mTBI.

There has also been increased research into psychological and social factors influencing PPCS, highlighting the role of factors such as pre-injury mental health difficulties (Ponsford et al., 2012), post-traumatic stress disorder (Lagarde et al., 2014; Porter et al., 2018), co-morbid anxiety and depression (Broshek et al., 2015) and the presence of post-injury litigation (Binder & Rohling, 1996; Carroll et al., 2004). The authors of this chapter are currently conducting a study into the influence of self-criticism on the development of PPCS in mTBI.

Theories of how PPCS is maintained have focused on misattributions of post-TBI symptoms, and expectations of recovery such as the "good old days" bias (Gunstad & Suhr, 2001), where people focus on how they think they were before the injury and become hypervigilant towards any perceived changes. The "expectation as aetiology" theory (Mittenberg et al., 1992) also highlights the importance of perceptions and beliefs about one's own symptoms. This is closely related to broader, well-established models within health psychology, such as the common-sense model of self-regulation (Leventhal et al., 1997), which highlight the cognitive and emotional processes driving threats to health. Such theories underline the importance of psychological assessment and formulation to understand cognitive and emotional processes within PPCS, as opposed to a sole focus on injury-related factors, such as the severity or mechanism of injury. However the aetiology of PPCS is defined, functional and organic neurological presentations can be equally disabling and distressing for patients and their families (Cope et al., 2017).

Clinical approaches to treatment

An mTBI expert group, including service user representation in Canada, has developed a comprehensive list of PPCS treatment guidelines based predominantly on clinical experience, but supported by limited evidence (Marshall et al., 2015). These guidelines advocate symptomatic treatment, including pharmacological treatment of headaches, and rehabilitation strategies for continued cognitive difficulties. However, treating individual symptoms may not be the most effective approach given the complex interplay between physical, emotional and cognitive factors.

In terms of psychological interventions, inconsistent research findings and methodological limitations hinder the development of clear guidance for effective treatments. A recent Cochrane review (Moore et al., 2019) indicated that cognitive-behavioural therapy (CBT), psychoeducation and cognitive rehabilitation may be effective, although good-quality evidence is limited. Some studies have reported on the effectiveness of psychological intervention in the first few weeks following mTBI, to influence expectations and perceptions of recovery, as a preventative approach to PPCS development (Alves et al., 1993; Wade et al., 1998). In their systematic review, Miller and Mittenberg (1998) reported on the effectiveness of a single psychoeducation session in preventing the development of, or reducing the duration of, PPCS. However, the effectiveness of information giving, education and reassurance alone for those experiencing PPCS was questioned in a more recent systematic review due to a lack of high-quality PPCS treatment studies (Al Sayegh et al., 2010).

Despite being the most researched PPCS treatment approach, limitations of CBT have been noted. A therapeutic focus on challenging "negative" thoughts is not always useful or appropriate to enable clinical change, especially within the context of identified physical or cognitive difficulties (Gilbert, 2009). People experiencing PPCS may feel defensive if they think a practitioner is implying that the (very real) physical symptoms they are experiencing are underpinned by psychological processes; this can reduce engagement in therapy. Therefore, a normalising and acceptance-based approach such as acceptance and commitment therapy (ACT) would, theoretically, be beneficial (Kangas & McDonald, 2011). ACT and mindfulness techniques can be helpful in coping with anxiety and stress – this may be of particular relevance within PPCS management if symptoms which are maintained by anxiety and stress can be alleviated through using these techniques (Bedard et al., 2003, 2014; Detert & Douglas, 2018).

Is ACT effective in mTBI and PPCS? The research evidence

The paucity of high-quality research into PPCS treatments across the board also applies to ACT (Al Sayegh et al., 2010; Bergersen et al., 2017). However, an emerging body of relevant research/case study evidence lends support to the effectiveness of ACT interventions in working with people with neurological presentations.

One ACT study and two reporting on mindfulness-based interventions were included in the recent Cochrane review (Moore et al., 2019), reporting no significant effects in comparison to controls (Bay et al., 2016; Bomyea et al., 2017; McMillan et al., 2002). However, a mindfulness-based stress reduction (MBSR) programme (another "third-wave" CBT-based intervention like ACT, which encompasses some of the same core elements, but without the emphasis on wider life values) did yield clinically meaningful effects on quality of life and self-efficacy in PPCS. The authors in this study postulated that effects resulted from acceptance and improved awareness, elements which overlap with core principles of ACT (Azulay et al., 2013). MBSR has also been effective in reducing depression and anxiety symptoms and improving coping in a mixed sample of functional and neurological presentations (Detert & Douglas, 2018).

Although not focused on PPCS specifically, Roche (2020) describes a case study highlighting the value of an ACT approach to managing post-traumatic stress disorder following TBI.

Furthermore, ACT and mindfulness-based interventions have been proposed as effective in other "medically unexplained" neurological presentations such as functional movement disorders, psychogenic non-epileptic seizures and symptoms associated with post-stroke anxiety (Barrett-Naylor et al., 2018; Baslet & Hill, 2011; Baslet et al., 2014; Cope et al., 2017; Graham et al., 2014, 2017). More broadly, there is a growing body of research supporting ACT interventions in non-neurological medically unexplained presentations including chronic pain (Hann & McCracken, 2014; McCracken & Vowles, 2014), irritable bowel syndrome (Gaylord et al., 2011) and somatisation (Lakhan & Schofield, 2013).

ACT approaches which focus on coping with and learning to tolerate unpleasant thoughts, feelings and sensations, as opposed to trying to challenge or fix them, could be a particularly good fit in working with medically unexplained presentations. By shifting the attention away from the struggle with difficult thoughts, feelings or sensations (i.e. not getting caught up in challenging them), a person can be supported to focus on making steps towards a more meaning-filled, values-based life.

Findings from the clinic room

The small but growing body of research evidence supporting ACT is consistent with the authors' experiences in the clinic room when treating PPCS. Working in a neurosciences centre doing lots of neuropsychological assessments with people who have experienced TBI can sometimes detract from our role and expertise as therapists. The authors therefore enjoyed attending an excellent introductory training on ACT (facilitated by Ray Owen), and reading Russ Harris's accessible introductory text, now in its second edition (Harris, 2019). Learning about ACT has revolutionised our therapy practice, and yielded palpable (albeit anecdotal) improvements in clinical outcomes across our caseloads, particularly when working with people who present with PPCS.

Our outcome measure of value is the visceral connection felt in the room; people nodding along with us; the two-handed sincere handshakes often received after initial sessions, and people reporting how helpful it has been to discuss the symptoms being experienced. We have come to realise how important it is for people experiencing PPCS to be heard and to be believed, and for a psychologically informed explanation to be given which builds on the person's understanding rather than dismisses their experiences. Many initial sessions have ended with mutual agreements of no further input being required, with people feeling reassured and confident to proceed with their life. The elements of ACT the authors have found particularly helpful in achieving such fruitful and clinically satisfying outcomes are as follows.

The initial session

Within many neuropsychology or neuroscience departments that cover a large geographical footprint, people may have to travel a long way to attend a session – this is often complicated by caring responsibilities, financial pressures and physical or cognitive impairments. Therefore, the finding that one session of psychoeducation (delivered early post-injury) could yield positive effects on reducing PPCS development (Alves et al., 1993) is useful to bear in mind; we can offer something useful in one meeting, even if the person is not able to attend for multiple sessions or extended psychological therapy.

Therefore, we suggest that the therapist's job in the first session is two-fold: to engage the person and normalise their experiences, and to educate about PPCS and its normal neuropsychological underpinnings. Interweaving the psychoeducative elements of initial PPCS intervention, within the backdrop of the ACT model in order to achieve these two aims, has been found by the authors to be particularly well received, and feels clinically effective and meaningful.

However, people who present with PPCS, may (understandably) feel defensive about being referred to a psychologist. They may feel that they are being told their symptoms are "all in their head" when they are experiencing palpable and disabling difficulties. In our experience, an ACT-congruent style facilitates initial engagement immeasurably by offering empathy and understanding about how we are all psychologically fallible, that we are all mere humans and that we are all the same. The ACT "two mountains" (Harris, 2019) analogy (communicating that we're all in it together) is a beautiful leveller, facilitating warmth and engagement.

Normalising PPCS development following mTBI, citing prevalence data to underline commonality, is crucial. Doing so, whilst noting how our minds are doing their usual protective "caveman" job warning us of danger (as all minds do), but with the volume turned up because something difficult/dangerous has recently happened, is a useful melding of PPCS/trauma information and ACT. Saying something like "you are not a robot: nobody could have suffered this trauma (with all of the scary thoughts about what might have happened) without experiencing some psychological symptoms" can be hugely beneficial.

Watching Russ Harris' excellent series of short YouTube animations is an efficient use of time in the first session to communicate difficult concepts clearly, palatably and quickly. The animation: *The Happiness Trap: Evolution of the Human Mind* (Harris, 2017) works particularly well in the first session of a PPCS intervention.

Within the second "first-session" task, regarding psychoeducation on PPCS, it can be useful to outline that while early symptoms may have been organic in nature, persistent symptoms are likely to be psychologically mediated. Psychological processes such as hypervigilance can heighten awareness of and exacerbate physical and cognitive symptoms such as pain or poor attention. It is not about saying that these processes are solely caused by psychological or emotional experiences, nor is it about saying that these processes are solely caused by neurological damage; it is about highlighting the impact that interactions between factors can have (think "both/and" rather than "either/or").

Experiential avoidance can be a useful concept to consider here, as many people with PPCS have developed unhelpful habits of avoiding difficult tasks. People experiencing PPCS, in the authors' experience, find it helpful to understand that the initial trauma and subsequent (understandable) experiential avoidance have contributed to prolonged (physical and cognitive) symptoms. It can be useful to emphasise that the mind and body are not separate, and that PPCS is a common problem following mTBI, experienced by many people. The YouTube animation *Headstuck! What is Experiential Avoidance?* (Harris, 2014) explains meaningfully and succinctly how we understandably fall into patterns of avoidance, reinforcing beliefs about not being able to cope. For example, if someone has been off work since their injury, they may be focused on not being able to do any aspect of their job. This might feel overwhelming – they may feel like a failure, that they are broken or that they are stuck. Discussing this in the context of experiential avoidance may be useful in helping them to consider what parts of the job they may be able to do again, what support they might need for other tasks and what they might need to approach differently – using trial and error, within a graded return to work. Some human self-disclosure (e.g. in the case of the first author, about often welling up whilst watching this animation) helps to cultivate strong, authentic therapeutic alliances.

It is also helpful to outline at the outset that PPCS can be responsive to ACT intervention in a number of ways: reconnecting with what's important in life and committing to actions in line with this (while symptoms may continue) can restore a sense of normality and purpose. Furthermore, it can be useful to share a formulation about the distracting nature of worrisome thoughts and how this reduces "brain space", thus causing cognitive mistakes. In turn, this strengthens fears about cognitive failings. Integrating this with what the person has talked about in the session can offer hope and support problem solving, while augmenting understanding of PPCS maintenance.

Ongoing therapeutic work

Where further therapeutic input is indicated/desired, particular aspects of ACT have proven fruitful when working with people presenting with PPCS. Empathic listening to the person's story; living the ACT model outside of the clinic room; humanness; use of humour; and appropriate self-disclosure of the therapist's own in vivo unwanted thoughts ("you're a crummy psychologist, yakking on about cavemen to people who have been through an awful experience") feel valuable and meaningful. Attending a monthly ACT peer supervision group with other psychologists also supports our clinical practice by enabling space for case discussion, reflecting on books we have read and training events we have attended. We also use experiential exercises to facilitate reflection and our willingness to "sit in the other chair".

Using physical gestures – like miming a hand talking away behind your head to illustrate our chattering minds – and effortfully miming "pushing a beach ball under the water" to illustrate the futility of emotional control can also authentically communicate that therapists are fully invested in the session and in connecting with the person in the room. Anecdotal service user feedback often highlights the value of authenticity and genuineness, and is sometimes contrasted with encounters with other health professionals.

Metaphors and analogies can be among the most powerful tools available to an ACT practitioner. As global intellectual ability is usually not compromised following mTBI, the large suite of helpful general ACT metaphors and exercises are all applicable. Our favourites include: "Thank you mind" (defusion); the 80th-birthday party speech (for identifying values);

and dropping anchor to help connect to the present moment (see Harris, 2019, for more examples). These can be useful in supporting willingness and acceptance of difficult thoughts, feelings or symptoms – by reducing the cognitive and emotional burden of the "struggle" with negative thoughts, feelings and symptoms and moving towards a place of acceptance (as in, willingness to accept difficult experiences), we have found that many people report that the severity of their symptoms is reduced. While symptom reduction is not a core aim within ACT per se and we would typically encourage focus on psychological flexibility and connection with valued activity, we believe that many people with PPCS could also find that physical and cognitive symptoms are indirectly alleviated through these approaches.

Sleep intervention

People who present with PPCS often report poor sleep, which inevitably amplifies cognitive slips, unwanted thoughts and emotional concerns. We have observed clinical benefits from learning about and practising the ACT-informed self-help sleep intervention proposed by Meadows (2014); this can be usefully integrated into a wider piece of work around coping, adjustment and supporting wellbeing.

Within this approach, many sleep hygiene tips (e.g. a warm bath before bed; lavender on the pillow; gentle music playing) are conceptualised as avoidance strategies – to avoid the uncomfortable thoughts and feelings experienced whilst lying in the dark when the thoughts flood in (a little like the beach ball bursting out of the water). The book poses the question "what do good sleepers do to get to sleep?" with the answer of course being – nothing! They just lie there. This can be a helpful perspective to adopt when working with people who have tried various sleep hygiene approaches and found little use in them – shifting the focus away from "trying" can reduce the frustration that often occurs. Employing ACT strategies whilst lying in bed can be a helpful vehicle to learning acceptance and defusion techniques, towards a hugely rewarding goal (better sleep), success in which has proven very beneficial in our clinical work with people experiencing PPCS.

Conclusion

There is a clear rationale for the value of ACT approaches in supporting people to manage and overcome PPCS, although currently there is a lack of empirical support to our anecdotal findings. The authors' experiences depict satisfying and efficacious work within the ACT model with people experiencing PPCS. We urge invested clinicians to contribute to high-quality research studies in this area, and to employ practice-based evidence, using approaches that feel helpful in the clinic room.

Suggested further reading

King, N. (2015). *Overcoming mild traumatic brain injury and post-concussion symptoms: A self-help guide using evidence-based techniques.* Robinson.

Meadows, G. (2014). *The sleep book: How to sleep well every night.* Orion.

Moore, P., Atherton, M. J., Wilson, J. A., & Jackson, C. (2019). Psychological interventions for persistent post-concussion symptoms following traumatic brain injury. *Cochrane Database of Systematic Reviews,* (3). https://doi.org/10.1002/14651858.cd012755

References

Al Sayegh, A., Sandford, D., & Carson, A. J. (2010). Psychological approaches to treatment of postconcussion syndrome: A systematic review. *Journal of Neurology, Neurosurgery & Psychiatry, 81*(10). https://doi.org/10.1136/jnnp.2008.170092

Alves, W., Macciocchi, S. N., & Barth, J. T. (1993). Postconcussive symptoms after uncomplicated mild head injury. *Journal of Head Trauma Rehabilitation, 8*(3), 48–59. https://doi.org/10.1097/00001199-199309000-00007

Azulay, J., Smart, C. M., Mott, T., & Cicerone, K. D. (2013). A pilot study examining the effect of mindfulness-based stress reduction on symptoms of chronic mild traumatic brain injury/postconcussive syndrome. *Journal of Head Trauma Rehabilitation, 28*(4), 323–331. https://doi.org/10.1097/htr.0b013e318250ebda

Barrett-Naylor, R., Gresswell, D. M., & Dawson, D. L. (2018). The effectiveness and acceptability of a guided self-help acceptance and commitment therapy (ACT) intervention for psychogenic nonepileptic seizures. *Epilepsy & Behavior,* 88, 332–340. https://doi.org/10.1016/j.yebeh.2018.09.039

Baslet, G., Dworetzky, B., Perez, D. L., & Ozer, M. (2014). Treatment of psychogenic nonepileptic seizures: Updated review and findings from a mindfulness-based intervention case series. *Clinical EEG and Neuroscience, 46*(1), 56–64. https://doi.org/10.1177/1550059414557025

Baslet, G., & Hill, J. (2011). Case report: Brief mindfulness-based psychotherapeutic intervention during inpatient hospitalization in a patient with conversion and dissociation. *Clinical Case Studies, 10*(2), 95–109. https://doi.org/10.1177/1534650110396359

Bay, E., Ribbens-Grimm, C., & Chan, R. R. (2016). Development and testing of two lifestyle interventions for persons with chronic mild-to-moderate traumatic brain injury: Acceptability and feasibility. *Applied Nursing Research, 30,* 90–93. https://doi.org/10.1016/j.apnr.2015.11.003

Bedard, M., Felteau, M., Marshall, S., Cullen, N., Gibbons, C., Dubois, S., Maxwell, H., Mazmanian, D., Weaver, B., Rees, L., Gainer, R., Klein, R., & Moustgaard, A. (2014). Mindfulness-based cognitive therapy reduces symptoms of depression in people with a traumatic brain injury: Results from a randomized controlled trial. *The Journal of Head Trauma Rehabilitation, 29*(4), 13–22. https://doi.org/10.1097/htr.0b013e3182a615a0

Bedard, M., Felteau, M., Mazmanian, D., Fedyk, K., Klein, R., Richardson, J., Parkinson, W., & Minthorn-Biggs, M.B. (2003). Pilot evaluation of a mindfulness-based intervention to improve quality of life among individuals who sustained traumatic brain injuries. *Disability and Rehabilitation, 25*(13), 722–731. https://doi.org/10.1080/0963828031000090489

Bergersen, K., Halvorsen, J. Ø., Tryti, E. A., Taylor, S. I., & Olsen, A. (2017). A systematic literature review of prolonged symptoms after mild traumatic brain injury. *Brain Injury, 31*(3), 279–289. https://doi.org/10.1080/02699052.2016.1255779

Binder, L. M., & Rohling, M. L. (1996). Money matters: A meta-analytic review of the effects of financial incentives on recovery after closed-head injury. *The American Journal of Psychiatry, 153*(1), 7–10. https://doi.org/10.1097/00001199-199608000-00012

Boake, C., McCauley, S. R., Levin, H. S., Pedroza, C., Contant, C. F., Song, J. X., … Diaz-Marchan, P. J. (2005). Diagnostic criteria for postconcussional syndrome after mild to moderate traumatic brain injury. *The Journal of Neuropsychiatry and Clinical Neurosciences, 17*(3), 350–356. https://doi.org/10.1176/jnp.17.3.350

Bomyea, J., Lang, A. J., & Schnurr, P. P. (2017). TBI and treatment response in a randomized trial of acceptance and commitment therapy. *Journal of Head Trauma Rehabilitation, 32*(5), E35–E43. https://doi.org/10.1097/htr.0000000000000278

Broshek, D. K., De Marco, A. P., & Freeman, J. R. (2015). A review of post-concussion syndrome and psychological factors associated with concussion. *Brain Injury, 29*(2), 228–237. https://doi.org/10.3109/02699052.2014.974674

Carroll, L. J., Cassidy, J. D., Peloso, P. M., Borg, J., von Holst, H., Holm, L., … Pepin, M. (2004). Prognosis for mild traumatic brain injury: Results of the WHO Collaborating Centre Task Force on Mild Traumatic Brain Injury. *Journal of Rehabilitation Medicine* (43 Suppl), 84–105. https://doi.org/10.1080/16501960410023859

Cope, S. R., Poole, N., & Agrawal, N. (2017). Treating functional non-epileptic attacks – Should we consider acceptance and commitment therapy? *Epilepsy & Behavior, 73*, 197–203. https://doi.org/10.1016/j.yebeh.2017.06.003

Dean, P. J. A., O'Neill, D., & Sterr, A. (2012). Post-concussion syndrome: Prevalence after mild traumatic brain injury in comparison with a sample without head injury. *Brain Injury, 26*(1), 14–26. https://doi.org/10.3109/02699052.2011.635354

Detert, N., & Douglas, L. (2018). Mindfulness MBSR/MBCT in a UK public health neurological service: Depression, anxiety, and perceived stress outcomes in a heterogeneous clinical sample of ninety-eight patients with neurological or functional neurological disorders. In G. Yeates & G. Farrell (Eds.), *Eastern influences on neuropsychotherapy: Accepting, soothing and stilling cluttered and critical minds* (pp. 211–232). Routledge.

Dunn, J. T., Lees-Haley, P. R., Brown, R. S., Williams, C. W., & English, L. T. (1995). Neurotoxic complaint base rates of personal injury claimants: Implications for neuropsychological assessment. *Journal of Clinical Psychology*, 51(4), 577–584. https://doi.org/10.1002/1097-4679(199507)51:4%3C577::aid-jclp2270510418%3E3.0.co;2-e

Gaylord, S., Palsson, O., Garland, E., Faurot, K., Coble, R., Mann, D., Frey, W., Leniek, K., & Whitehead, W. (2011). Mindfulness training reduces the severity of irritable bowel syndrome in women: Results of a randomized controlled trial. *American Journal of Gastroenterology, 106*(9), 1678–1688. https://doi.org/10.1038/ajg.2011.184

Gilbert, P. (2009). *The compassionate mind.* New Harbinger.

Graham, C. D., Gillanders, D., Stuart, S., & Gouick, J. (2014). An acceptance and commitment therapy (ACT)-based intervention for an adult experiencing post-stroke anxiety and medically unexplained symptoms. *Clinical Case Studies, 14*(2), 83–97. https://doi.org/10.1177/1534650114539386

Graham, C. D., Stuart, S. R., O'Hara D. J., & Kemp, S. (2017). Using acceptance and commitment therapy to improve outcomes in functional movement disorders: A case study. *Clinical Case Studies, 16*(5), 401–416. https://doi.org/10.1177/1534650117706544

Gunstad, J., & Suhr, J. A. (2001). 'Expectation as etiology' versus 'the good old days': Postconcussion syndrome symptom reporting in athletes, headache sufferers, and depressed individuals. *Journal of the International Neuropsychological Society: JINS, 7*(3), 323–333. https://doi.org/10.1017/s1355617701733061

Hann, K. E. J., & McCracken, L. M. (2014). A systematic review of randomized controlled trials of acceptance and commitment therapy for adults with chronic pain: Outcome domains, design quality, and efficacy. *Journal of Contextual Behavioral Science, 3*(4), 217–227. https://doi.org/10.1016/j.jcbs.2014.10.001

Harris, R. (2014). *Headstuck! What is experiential avoidance?* [Video]. Youtube. www.youtube.com/watch?v=C-ZuqeyxULM

Harris, R. (2017). *The happiness trap: Evolution of the human mind.* [Video]. Youtube. www.youtube.com/watch?v=kv6HkipQcfA

Harris, R. (2019). *ACT made simple: A quick-start guide to ACT basics and beyond* (2nd ed.). New Harbinger.

Hellstrøm, T., Westlye, L. T., Kaufmann, T., Nhat Trung, D., Søberg, H. L., Sigurdardottir, S. … Andelic, N. (2017). White matter microstructure is associated with functional, cognitive, and emotional symptoms 12 months after mild traumatic brain injury. *Scientific Reports, 7*(1), 13795. https://doi.org/10.1038/s41598-017-13628-1

Iverson, G. L. (2006). Misdiagnosis of the persistent postconcussion syndrome in patients with depression. *Archives of Clinical Neuropsychology: The Official Journal of the National Academy of Neuropsychologists, 21*(4), 303–310. https://doi.org/10.1016/j.acn.2005.12.008

Iverson, G. L., & Lange, R. T. (2003). Examination of 'postconcussion-like' symptoms in a healthy sample. *Applied Neuropsychology, 10*(3), 137–144. https://doi.org/10.1207/s15324826an1003_02

Kangas, M., & McDonald, S. (2011). Is it time to ACT? The potential of acceptance and commitment therapy for psychological problems following acquired brain injury. *Neuropsychological Rehabilitation,* 21(2), 250–276. https://doi.org/10.1080/09602011.2010.540920

Lagarde, E., Salmi, L.-R., Holm, L. W., Contrand, B., Masson, F., Ribéreau-Gayon, R., … Cassidy, J. D. (2014). Association of symptoms following mild traumatic brain injury with posttraumatic stress disorder vs postconcussion syndrome. *JAMA Psychiatry, 71*(9), 1032–1040. https://doi.org/10.1001/jamapsychiatry.2014.666

Lakhan, S. E., & Schofield, K. M. (2013). Mindfulness-based therapies in the treatment of somatization disorders: A systematic review and meta-analysis. *PLoS One, 8*(8), e71834. https://doi.org/10.1371/journal.pone.0071834

Lannsjo, M., af Geijerstam, J.-L., Johansson, U., Bring, J., & Borg, J. (2009). Prevalence and structure of symptoms at 3 months after mild traumatic brain injury in a national cohort. *Brain Injury, 23*(3), 213–219. https://doi.org/10.1080/02699050902748356

Leventhal, H., Benyamini, Y., Brownlee, S., Diefenbach, M., Leventhal, E. A., & Patrick-Miller, L. (1997). Illness representations: Theoretical foundations. In K. J. Petrie & J. A. Weinman (Eds.), *Perceptions of health and illness: Current research and applications* (pp. 19–45). Harwood Academic Publishers.

Marshall, S., Bayley, M., McCullagh, S., Velikonja, D., Berrigan, L., Ouchterlony, D., & Weegar, K. (2015). Updated clinical practice guidelines for concussion/mild traumatic brain injury and persistent symptoms. *Brain Injury, 29*(6), 688–700. https://doi.org/10.3109/02699052.2015.1004755

McCracken, L. M., & Vowles, K. E. (2014). Acceptance and commitment therapy and mindfulness for chronic pain: Model, process, and progress. *American Psychologist, 69*, 178–187. https://doi.org/10.1037/a0035623

McCrea, M. A. (2008). *Mild traumatic brain injury and postconcussion syndrome: The new evidence base for diagnosis and treatment.* Oxford University Press.

McMillan, T., Robertson, I. H., Brock, D., & Chorlton, L. (2002). Brief mindfulness training for attentional problems after traumatic brain injury: A randomised control treatment trial. *Neuropsychological Rehabilitation, 12*(2), 117–125. https://doi.org/10.1080/09602010143000202

Meadows, G. (2014). *The sleep book: How to sleep well every night.* Orion.

Miller, L. J., & Mittenberg, W. (1998). Brief cognitive behavioral interventions in mild traumatic brain injury. *Applied Neuropsychology*, 5(4), 172–183. https://doi.org/10.1207/s15324826an0504_2

Mittenberg, W., DiGiulio, D. V., Perrin, S., & Bass, A. E. (1992). Symptoms following mild head injury: Expectation as aetiology. *Journal of Neurology, Neurosurgery, and Psychiatry*, 55(3), 200–204. https://doi.org/10.1136/jnnp.55.3.200

Moore, P., Atherton, M. J., Wilson, J. A., & Jackson, C. (2019). Psychological interventions for persistent post-concussion symptoms following traumatic brain injury. *Cochrane Database of Systematic Reviews*, 3. https://doi.org/10.1002/14651858.cd012755

National Institute for Health and Care Excellence (NICE). (2019). *Head injury: Assessment and early management, Clinical guideline 176.* www.nice.org.uk/guidance/cg176

Polinder, S., Cnossen, M. C., Real, R. G. L., Covic, A., Gorbunova, A., Voormolen, D. C., ... von Steinbuechel, N. (2018). A multidimensional approach to post-concussion symptoms in mild traumatic brain injury. *Frontiers in Neurology, 9*, 1113. https://doi.org/10.3389/fneur.2018.01113

Ponsford, J., Cameron, P., Fitzgerald, M., Grant, M., Mikocka-Walus, A., & Schonberger, M. (2012). Predictors of postconcussive symptoms 3 months after mild traumatic brain injury. *Neuropsychology, 26*(3), 304–313. https://doi.org/10.1037/a0027888

Porter, K. E., Stein, M. B., Martis, B., Avallone, K. M., McSweeney, L. B., Smith, E. R., ... Rauch, S. A. M. (2018). Postconcussive symptoms (PCS) following combat-related traumatic brain injury (TBI) in veterans with posttraumatic stress disorder (PTSD): Influence of TBI, PTSD, and depression on symptoms measured by the Neurobehavioral Symptom Inventory (NSI). *Journal of Psychiatric Research, 102*, 8–13. https://doi.org/10.1016/j.jpsychires.2018.03.004

Radanov, B. P., Dvorak, J., & Valach, L. (1992). Cognitive deficits in patients after soft tissue injury of the cervical spine. *Spine, 17*(2), 127–131. https://doi.org/10.1097/00007632-199202000-00001

Reuben, A., Sampson, P., Harris, A. R., Williams, H., & Yates, P. (2014). Postconcussion syndrome (PCS) in the emergency department: Predicting and pre-empting persistent symptoms following a mild traumatic brain injury. *Emergency Medicine Journal: EMJ, 31*(1), 72–77. https://doi.org/10.1136/emermed-2012-201667

Richter, S., Winzeck, S., & Kornaropoulos, E. N. (2021). Neuroanatomical substrates and symptoms associated with magnetic resonance imaging of patients with mild traumatic brain injury. *JAMA Network Open, 4*(3), e210994. https://doi.org/10.1001/jamanetworkopen.2021.0994

Roche, L. (2020). An acceptance and commitment therapy-based intervention for PTSD following traumatic brain injury: A case study. *Brain Injury, 34*(2), 290–297. https://doi.org/10.1080/02699052.2019.1683896

Silverberg, N. D., & Iverson, G. L. (2011). Etiology of the post-concussion syndrome: Physiogenesis and psychogenesis revisited. *Neurorehabilitation, 29*(4), 317–329. https://doi.org/10.3233/nre-2011-0708

Teasdale, G., & Jennett, B. (1974). Assessment of coma and impaired consciousness: A practical scale. *Lancet, 2*(7872), 81–84. https://doi.org/10.1016/s0140-6736(74)91639-0

Wade, D., King, N., Wenden, F., Crawford, S., & Caldwell, F. (1998). Routine follow-up after head injury: A second randomised controlled trial. *Journal of Neurology, Neurosurgery & Psychiatry, 65*(2), 177–183. https://doi.org/10.1136/jnnp.65.2.177

Acceptance and commitment therapy for people with moderate or severe brain injuries

Emma Cameron, Mark A. Oliver and Will Curvis

Abstract

People with moderate or severe brain injuries often experience cognitive problems, language and communication impairments and physical or sensory changes. These difficulties can complicate the rehabilitation and adjustment journey. Acceptance and commitment therapy (ACT) has the potential to be adapted for use with people who have experienced moderate or severe brain injuries and their families/carers, to support neuropsychological rehabilitation and emotional adjustment. Stepping away from language-heavy metacognitive activities and considering how to increase a person's ability to process and consolidate information, along with focusing on committed actions towards longer-term goals, might help to maximise engagement in rehabilitation, goal setting and goal attainment.

Brain injuries exist on a spectrum of severity. Different classification systems exist to help clinicians gauge the severity of injury and likely impairments based on variables such as initial eye, verbal and motor responses, length of loss of consciousness/coma or length of post-traumatic amnesia (Rabinowitz & Levin, 2014; Ruttan et al., 2008). Moderate or severe brain injuries are typically associated with more significant and longer-lasting physical, cognitive, communication and emotional problems (Lippert-Grüner et al., 2006; Rabinowitz & Levin, 2014; Ruttan et al., 2008).

Different areas of the brain are associated with different functions; when damage occurs to a specific region of the brain, changes in these functions are likely. However, the human brain is highly complex and even the simplest behavioural function or emotional response is the result of interplay between a variety of different anatomical pathways, systems and connections; therefore, a brain injury can lead to a wide range of symptoms. After the initial injury, secondary problems such as hydrocephalus and seizures can develop, potentially leading to further localised or general damage to the brain.

Physical impairments following moderate or severe brain injury can lead to difficulties with gait or mobility; this may involve weakness or paralysis

DOI: 10.4324/9781003024408-8

of limbs (either complete, or of one side of the body) or coordination issues. Fatigue is often a problem. Changes to sensory input processing and sensation are common, with many people experiencing visual problems (such as visual field loss or agnosia), or issues with hearing, smell, touch, taste or proprioception. Severe injuries can result in impaired respiratory function, sometimes requiring insertion of a tracheostomy which may be acute or long-term. Communication problems can include receptive aphasia (difficulties with comprehension of written/spoken language) and/or expressive aphasia (difficulties with language production).

Cognitive problems are also common, including difficulties within domains such as visual and verbal memory, attention, processing speed, language, visual processing (e.g. spatial awareness, object perception, facial perception, visual neglect) and executive functioning (a group of skills encompassing, amongst others, planning, initiating, inhibition, decision making, flexibility, self-awareness and self-monitoring). A full and thorough description of the sequelae of moderate or severe brain injury is beyond the scope of this chapter; for an accessible overview see Morgan and Ricker (2008) and Newby et al. (2013).

Although there are no absolute rules, more severe brain injuries are typically associated with more severe physical, cognitive and communication impairments. These difficulties may require a period of acute hospital-based care or inpatient rehabilitation (especially if the brain injury is severe enough to cause a prolonged disorder of consciousness). The person may require support with completing simple activities of daily living (e.g. washing and dressing) or their needs may be around functional or vocational rehabilitation (e.g. considering adaptations needed for living independently or a return to employment). Trajectories of recovery following severe brain injury are highly variable; some people may make a full physical and/or neuropsychological recovery, while others may require professional 24-hour care or support from family/carers with activities of daily living for the rest of their lives.

These changes and challenges mean a potentially difficult period of adjustment and acceptance for the individual and their family. The psychological sequelae of suffering a moderate or severe brain injury can include depression, anxiety, irritability and aggressiveness, both in the immediate aftermath of the injury and for years afterwards (Doering & Exner, 2011), with over half of people meeting criteria for major depressive disorder a year after injury (Bombardier et al., 2010). The psychosocial consequences can include the loss of roles, hobbies, interests, social interactions and independence (Morton & Wehman, 1995). Typically, more severe impairments are associated with higher levels of emotional distress (Ciurli et al., 2011; Jorge et al., 2007; Rabinowitz & Levin, 2014). Significant functional disability caused by physical or cognitive impairments often leads to grief and anxiety, as part of a process of psychosocial adjustment and identity change (Beadle et al., 2016). This process can be complicated by issues around insight, awareness or other cognitive problems (van der Horn et al., 2013); a person is unlikely to be motivated to engage in painful and tiring physiotherapy sessions if they do not recognise that they have rehabilitation needs, which may have negative implications for their psychological wellbeing and physical recovery. Many of the challenges experienced by people who have experienced severe brain injuries are best understood as an interconnected constellation of physical, cognitive and psychological factors, occurring within a social context.

This highlights the importance of a biopsychosocial approach to neuro-psychological assessment and rehabilitation, incorporating emotional well-being as part of recovery outcomes. National guidance and standards for best practice highlight the importance of psychological input for people who have experienced brain injuries. However, neuropsychological and physical impairments can make traditionally delivered psychological therapies less accessible or available. Psychological services are often not set up to be particularly accessible to people with problems with fatigue, impaired motivation, awareness/insight, memory impairments or executive dysfunction. Cognitive impairments can stop someone from attending to, understanding or remembering the content of therapy sessions, especially with approaches such as cognitive-behavioural therapy (CBT) which typically involve homework tasks and carryover of information between sessions (Wong et al., 2012).

Acceptance and commitment therapy and psychological flexibility

As described elsewhere in this text, acceptance and commitment therapy (ACT) has attracted a great deal of research attention and has been usefully applied as a transdiagnostic approach across a range of settings, including supporting people with physical health problems (Bai et al., 2020; Gloster et al., 2020; Graham et al., 2016). ACT was developed out of relational frame theory (RFT), an operant account of verbal language that explains how language can exert influence over human behaviour, extending humans' capacity to learn far beyond our actual experience. RFT suggests it is linguistically impossible to have a "higher" without an implicit or explicit "lower"; no "better" without a "worse". However, the incalculable advantages inferred on human development by the ability to use complex language bring disadvantages. We experience pain and distress over things that have never happened, or that happened years ago. We become locked into cycles of rumination, crippled by regret, and compare ourselves unfavourably with the people around us. We spend the majority of our lives inside our heads, somewhat or considerably removed from the actual experience of our five senses (Hayes et al., 2001, 2012; Törneke, 2010).

ACT recognises the inevitable and universal nature of this suffering as part of the human condition. If we are psychologically rigid in the presence of challenging events or difficult emotions, we find ourselves pulled into our heads, away from the world as it is in this precise moment. We lose contact with the things that are important to us (Hayes et al., 2012). ACT therefore looks to increase psychological flexibility; if we can experience events, feelings, thoughts and sensations as they are – transient unpleasant experiences that may ebb and flow in their own time – they do not need to define us or restrict our lives.

Acceptance and commitment therapy for people with moderate or severe brain injuries

Although there is promising evidence supporting the use of ACT after brain injury, there is little research directly exploring the use of ACT for individuals with significant cognitive impairment (Kangas & McDonald, 2011). Most of the available research exploring use of ACT within brain injury focuses on the mild to moderate end of the spectrum (e.g. Bédard et al., 2003; Kangas & McDonald, 2011; Roemer et al., 2008) or does not differentiate by brain injury severity. This makes it difficult to draw firm conclusions about specific adaptations to ACT approaches for people with more severe brain injuries.

A small amount of research has explored how ACT might be adapted to meet the needs of other populations, for example people with intellectual disabilities (Byrne & O'Mahony, 2020). Pankey and Hayes (2003) reported a four-session ACT-based intervention to support medication provision with a woman with psychosis and intellectual disability. Brown and Hooper (2009) outlined an approach designed around mindfulness and ACT-based experiential activities, to support a client with an intellectual disability to learn to notice anxious thoughts and distance herself from their content. Oliver et al. (2019) reported two case studies, both showing rapid improvement in supporting two women with intellectual disabilities to manage distressing intrusive thoughts and strong emotions such as anger, using techniques around focused attention toward the present moment (including breath, sensory and object exercises) and reinforcement of moves towards valued living.

However, it remains somewhat unclear how these principles might be adapted to support people with acquired brain injuries. How do we explain an abstract concept to someone who struggles to understand and retain complex information? How can we help someone with memory and initiation problems to remember how and when they might use a technique? How do we promote psychological flexibility, when the cognitive ability to "think flexibly" may be impaired as part of the brain injury (Whiting et al., 2015)?

Adapting and applying ACT techniques

As severe brain injury can lead to long-term cognitive impairments (Tagliaferri et al., 2006), adaptations to psychological therapy are required, to reduce barriers that may be caused by attention, communication, memory and executive functioning difficulties. Gallagher et al. (2016) reviewed the literature around adaptations for delivering CBT for people with cognitive impairments following brain injury, highlighting the importance of practical strategies such as writing down homework tasks and using other memory aids. Soo et al. (2011) conducted a literature review around ACT and its applicability to people with acquired brain injury. They suggested that adaptations for the more "cognitive" components, such as cognitive defusion, were consistent with what might be found within other therapeutic approaches (e.g. repetition, pauses, summarising, use of written/pictorial aids). Drawing on the intellectual disability literature can also be useful; adaptations such as giving more time, simplifying or "chunking" information, use of non-verbal communication and supplementary materials (drawings, object use) are well-established adaptations for psychological therapy with people with intellectual disabilities (Banks, 2003; Surley & Dagnan, 2019). Focusing on direct experience, visual aids and structured worksheets may therefore be helpful for this population, if the nature of the impairments they experience permits them to make use of such strategies.

Information can be delivered in more than one modality and provided in a format that is relevant and meaningful to the individual, and helpful for both processing and remembering of information (Simpson et al., 2011; Westmacott & Moscovitch, 2003). People with severe brain injuries are also likely to require additional time and repetition to consolidate techniques or concepts; remember that few people in the general population find that ACT techniques and principles come naturally and are easily understood. Most core ACT protocols highlight the importance of regular practice between sessions. When introducing an idea or a technique to someone who has experienced brain injury, be prepared for understanding and consolidation to take additional time. Do not assume too quickly that someone is incapable of being able to do something. Stay curious about why a person might be struggling to put something into practice – could this reflect a memory impairment, or problems with initiation? Involvement of care staff or family members, either in attendance at sessions or supporting exercises outside of this, will be helpful.

Research has suggested that metaphor use improves understanding of challenging concepts for individuals with brain injuries and is useful for those with concrete thinking styles, poor working memory and slowed processing speed (Lakoff & Johnson, 1999; Ylvisaker et al., 2008) – though of course, "abstract" metaphors may prove too challenging for those with concrete thinking styles, and careful trial and error may be required. Strategic use of metaphors may also help to reduce reliance on verbal means of expression, key for those with moderate to severe brain injuries where language is more likely to be impacted (Rabinowitz & Levin, 2014).

Fundamentally, the emphasis is on being client-led – this should involve an in-depth initial assessment phase which involves establishing a person's level of ability and any neuropsychological, physical or sensory impairments, to ensure that any intervention work falls within a person's ability to understand and make use of the concepts or strategies being considered. It is also worth considering whether someone is able to: (1) describe what thoughts and feelings are; and (2) identify and reflect on their own thoughts, as this would most likely steer the extent to which the person would be able to engage in work around psychological flexibility. Although validation studies are in their infancy, the Psychological Flexibility Questionnaire – Accessible (PFQ-AX; Oliver, 2020) was designed to tap into the same constructs as existing measures of acceptance and cognitive fusion, in a more acceptable and accessible way with improved readability and simpler language. Preliminary data indicate that this measure may be useful in tracking changes in psychological flexibility in people with intellectual disabilities; as of yet, no studies have explored the use of this measure with people with severe brain injury.

A range of ACT-based exercises can be used to support psychological flexibility and cognitive defusion, based on the simplified core processes described by Harris (2019) of "Be present", "Open up" and "Do what matters". The suggestions below (based on the authors' clinical practice) are centred around the behavioural and experiential aspects of ACT, which are potentially more accessible than approaches based on verbal reasoning such as CBT. We do not propose them as being perfect or complete solutions; we hope they serve as a spark for your own creativity.

Be present

Attention and information-processing impairments are common after brain injury. Therefore, any exercises or techniques designed to focus on these skills must be carefully considered. Short exercises are likely to be more feasible – it may be useful to start with simple, concrete, structured mindful breathing or body-scanning-type exercises (e.g. a body outline with prompts of things to look for – such as "Where do you feel the emotion? Notice if you have tight shoulders, butterflies in your stomach … achy feet"). Audio/video recordings or smartphone apps are likely to work better then written instructions, as the person may struggle to read/remember instructions – there are lots of examples available for free on the internet, or the person may prefer to design something more personalised.

Some people – especially those with physical problems such as pain, mobility or breathing difficulties – may find externally focused exercises easier than those which draw attention to the body or internal sensations. Mindfulness exercises which encourage paying attention to the five senses (e.g. notice three things you can hear … notice three things you can smell) can be useful, but consideration should be given to any sensory impairments (e.g. visual/hearing impairments, reduced sense of smell) or sensory-processing problems (e.g. hypersensitivity). Focus on intact senses wherever possible – for example, someone with a visual impairment might still be able to hold an object in their hand and focus their attention that way, or they might be able to keep some food (e.g. a chocolate or raisin) in their mouth and notice the sensations as they hold their attention (though this may not be possible for those with impaired swallow abilities or those on modified diets). One of the authors (MO) worked with Rokaya,[1] a woman with visual impairment and intellectual disabilities. She found it difficult to unhook from her thoughts during mindfulness exercises. Although prompts were given, this was altogether too passive for Rokaya to follow. Directing Rokaya to do something active like pat her legs with her hands was cognitively demanding enough to pull her out of her thoughts and into the present moment.

As another example of joint attention on a present-moment awareness task, MO worked with Bill, a man with significant cognitive impairment who would get stuck in repetitive, ruminative cycles of assurance seeking that could never be answered to his satisfaction. He couldn't engage with eyes-closed mindfulness tasks for more than 3 seconds without seeking assurance, but when encouraged to maintain eye contact as both MO and Bill slowly counted to 20, joint attention on the present moment was possible. This provided a foundation for more complex defusion work.

It is also worth considering how to embed these "present-moment" exercises into a regular practice routine. Associations with everyday activities work well – for example, can the person practise focusing their attention on the sensations being experienced every time they brush their teeth, or do their washing up? External prompts such as reminders or alerts on a smartphone, tablet or smartwatch can also be set to provide a cue – this can act as a trigger to practise an exercise, or can be utilised as a more concrete "check-in" to bring the person's attention to the present moment – "where is your mind right now?" works well as a calendar alert on a smartphone or tablet. Recent advances in voice-controlled technology (such as Amazon's Alexa or the Google Assistant) open up a world of options for those with physical or sensory impairments, whether in setting up reminders, questions or triggering other applications such as music. WC once spent an interesting therapy session mindfully focusing in on the bass guitar riffs on a speed metal track chosen by the person he was working with (a keen musician). WC and the client listened to the track together for 30 seconds, then discussed what each person noticed about the notes being played, the volume and tone of the instrument at different times in the mix, how it was panned to the left and right channel of the stereo field, and so on – details that were only noticeable (to WC, at least) when attention was directed in this way. This served as a useful starting point for broader conversations about mindfulness-based activities and how shifting the spotlight of attention can be helpful.

Self-as-context is one of the more difficult ACT concepts to learn and to explain (Westrup, 2014) and so is often avoided by unsure clinicians. However, if successfully communicated, it can be one of the most powerful

ACT interventions. Self-as-context is the view of the self that transcends all of the stories, beliefs and labels we carry about ourselves – if we can hold all of these things lightly (the good and the bad, the true and the debatable), we are less likely to be led by them in unhelpful directions. After brain injury, these stories, beliefs and labels are likely to be very different to what they were before.

Various metaphors to help illustrate this are described in many introductory books on ACT; our suggestion would be to consider how you can make your metaphor understandable and validating to the person you are working with. For example, Harris (2019) describes the chessboard metaphor (in which we are neither the white pieces nor the black, but instead are the infinitely expansive board on which any number of combinations of plays can be enacted) – explanation of this could be supported by an actual chessboard. Discussing the container metaphor (in which you are the limitless container of all of your life's experiences) could be supported by a tub or container to fill with stones (or other items). The principles of "self-as-context" can be illustrated and made more experiential in lots of ways; for example, ask the individual (or their family) to bring in photographs of them at different life stages (as a baby, infant, child, teenager, adult). This might help to explore the idea that there is an observing self, distinct from our bodies that have been continuously changing, but always, continuously "you". This can be particularly pertinent following brain injury.

It can be even more powerful if a person generates their own metaphor or analogy. WC worked with Gill, who spoke about how her physical and cognitive impairments left her feeling like "a jigsaw, all messed up, with some of the puzzle pieces missing". This concept was captured by writing each element of the formulation on a picture of puzzle pieces, with each "piece" of the puzzle reflecting a different aspect of the self (e.g. worry about the future; pain; memory problems; relationship with partner). This provided a concrete way to discuss what element of the formulation we were focusing on at a particular moment (e.g. difficult thoughts and feelings) and to think about how different areas interacted. Later in the work, the jigsaw metaphor was used as part of conversations around identity and change – we talked about what pieces had changed since Gill's brain injury (memory, mobility) and what pieces had not (e.g. sense of humour, values, priorities in life). This opened up conversations about how focusing only on the pieces that were "missing" made it harder to step back and see the bigger picture that the jigsaw represented – if we had enough of the "right" pieces, we could still see the picture. Towards the end of the work, Gill also made the wonderful comment that her life was much more complex and flexible than a jigsaw that could only be put together in one singular, "correct" way. She decided that Lego was a better representation for her than a jigsaw, as although there might be an initial plan or design when you buy a Lego set, the real beauty of Lego is that it can be made into all kinds of different things.

This level of abstraction and complexity may be too much for some people and it may be necessary to focus on simpler elements – such as discussing aspects of the "self" that are the same or different before and after the injury. People can often feel that their whole identity changes to being a person with a brain injury or a disability; it can be helpful for the person to reflect on what sort of person they are, how others would describe them and what has stayed the same despite the brain injury. As discussed earlier, RFT considers verbal language a double-edged sword; if we cannot have "better" without "worse", it is incredibly difficult to think about current circumstances without thinking of how things were. Unpicking ideas around "the good old days" and considering how focus can be taken away from the present moment can be a useful therapeutic direction, if done in an empathic and validating manner.

Open up

Explaining concepts in simple language can present challenges for clinicians; there is no better test for how well we truly understand a concept than having to explain it without using jargon or technical terms. Metaphors can be useful – WC worked with Dave, who experienced a diffuse axonal injury in a road traffic accident. Showing Dave a picture of the wires in a computer helped him conceptualise how axonal damage could lead to "brain messages" not always getting to where they needed to be, which was why he struggled to remember things and his brain felt "slow". This metaphor also served as a useful foundation for Dave learning to notice his thoughts as part of a more abstract concept of the mind – "what's going through the wires right now?" Understanding the impact of his brain injury on his thinking skills, information-processing speed and emotional responses helped Dave to see these thoughts as "signals going through the wires" – this small but powerful shift was vital in supporting his acceptance of and ability to cope with difficult thoughts and emotions.

These principles can also guide how we help someone to make sense of defusion concepts and exercises. Help information processing, consolidation and recall by using meaningful images – e.g. instead of leaves on a stream you might use baggage on a luggage carousel or a busy high street with lots of people walking past. A video of trains pulling in and out of a station might serve as a useful way to talk about how thoughts can come and go – we can watch from the platform without getting on the train. The sound of the ocean's waves (rather than just a picture or description of waves) might be helpful in showing someone how thoughts and feelings ebb and flow, and how we can watch this from the shore without being swept up in the current. A football fan might be encouraged to imagine a player about to take a penalty kick at Wembley Stadium – they hear their own fans shouting encouraging (but distracting) comments, and fans of the opposition shouting much more critical or abusive things – a bit like how our minds throw positive and negative thoughts at us. A good footballer would not be able to ignore those distractions, but they might be able to notice them without being hooked by them.

If visualisation techniques around representing or externalising thoughts are too abstract or difficult to understand, be more concrete. WC recently asked a client to write a difficult thought on a piece of paper and balance it on her head for a minute, before then holding it on her lap. This helped to illustrate the difference between a thought being "fused" and "defused". The client then practised writing the thought in different-sized writing, and saying it out loud. Other defusion techniques based around externalising thoughts in this way (e.g. saying them in a silly voice, singing thoughts out loud) can be useful – though take care when working with people with speech/communication impairments, who may find this difficult.

Take care not to let techniques or exercises distract from the reason why you are introducing them. The whole focus of an intervention may be centred around making the point that thoughts are just thoughts – and we can engage with them in different ways.

Even this might be too much for people who are unable to identify or reflect on their thoughts. WC worked with Ryan during his rehabilitation, a man who experienced a very severe brain injury and was left with significant cognitive impairments. Ryan was highly perseverative and had limited language skills – he often got "stuck" saying things like "my brain is broken", which resulted in him becoming extremely distressed and upset for hours at a time. It was hard for anyone to calm him down or distract him from this pain – distraction did not help and giving him space to talk and perseverate seemed to keep him stuck. The interaction between his thoughts, feelings and the nature of his cognitive impairment kept him in a constant state of distress.

It was helpful to conceptualise this distress from an RFT perspective – we conceptualised the negative things Ryan was saying about himself as being reflective of his thoughts at that moment, even if he could not name them as "thoughts". Ryan's comments provided fairly good evidence that, although he might not have been able to reflect on his thought processes in a typical sense, Ryan was able to "relationally frame" – he knew that he was "worse" than before his injury. This reflected some emerging awareness of his impairments.

What seemed to help was an approach designed to validate first, and then gently reframe. When Ryan said "my brain is broken", WC responded by focusing on the emotions and asking Ryan how he felt about this – this usually got a one-word answer that we won't print here, but that gave good insight into how he felt. After doing some neuropsychological testing that suggested Ryan had a particularly short attentional/working-memory span, WC and the rehabilitation team began to respond to Ryan's comment "my brain is broken" by saying "yes – your brain can't do some things – but it can do some things just as well". Ryan began to repeat this, still in a perseverative way – "my brain is broken but it can do some things well" – however, he became significantly less distressed. Ryan began to repeat this back much more easily, using different words to make the same point. He was not simply repeating words verbatim; he was integrating the words into his thought processes, learning and remembering through this repetition. We quickly noticed that the periods of high distress were significantly reduced and he seemed much more positive throughout the day.

By intervening at a "language" level, were we able to shift what he experienced as internal thoughts? It is hard to say for sure, but Ryan seemed to benefit from this approach – loosely based around the concept of defusion – of reshaping and redirecting the thoughts by shifting attentional focus and creating space for other perspectives, without dismissing or invalidating the initial thoughts. The repetition seemed to help the more balanced thoughts "stick" in Ryan's mind more easily, and he became more able to generate these responses with fewer prompts from staff.

Do what matters

ACT focuses on facilitating functional change, and as goals for those with moderate to severe brain injuries tend to relate to helping people to re-engage in functional activities and living a meaningful life in spite of neurological deficits, this approach is well suited to the neurorehabilitation arena. Values are key in goal-setting theory (Locke & Latham, 1990). Exploration of values improves goal setting and goal attainment (e.g. Chase et al., 2013; Roemer et al., 2008).

Values exploration may therefore help individuals with severe brain injuries to engage in neurorehabilitation, where a significant barrier to engagement is purported to be poor self-identity or sense of self (Ylvisaker et al., 2008). Values-based work can help to build sense of self as values provide a common thread in the individual's pre- and post-brain injury self, helping them to "find themselves" during the adjustment process (e.g. Van Bost et al., 2017). Furthermore, as some studies have indicated that increased injury severity correlates with reduced functional outcomes (Ponsford et al., 2008), meaning individuals may not be able to return to previous "indicators" of their values (e.g. paid employment, role within the family), a shift from goals to values can be important to help re-evaluate how to move towards what is important to them, as part of the ongoing journey of adjustment. After all, adjustment is often not simply returning to life as it was – that may not be possible, but it might also not be what is wanted.

A common method of identifying values is using the personal values card sort task (Miller et al., 2001). This task seems well suited to those with significant cognitive impairment post-brain injury as it provides values in a concrete manner on printed cards, which are then sorted into three piles: "not important to me", "important to me" and "very important to me". As those with significant cognitive deficits after brain injury can struggle with information processing, attention, evaluation/judgement and decision making, utilising shorter methods is prudent to ensure the person can fully engage with the task within the timeframe of a session. Harris (2020) provides a set with pictures; however there is still a large amount of text on each card, including long/complex words. Some adapted personal values card sorts have already been suggested in the neurorehabilitation community. For example, Winson et al. (2017) utilised the original 83 values cards, but reduced the amount of cognitive load by reducing the information provided on each card. There are many free lists of values available online which can be adapted or simplified, considering the person's sensory, physical and cognitive needs. This exercise can also be supported by printing out in large letters the titles for each pile (e.g. very important, quite important, not important) to reduce burdens on memory.

There are many ways to prompt reflection on values. Boulton et al. (2018) reported on a six-session feasibility study exploring if adults with intellectual disabilities could utilise photography to help them clarify their values. People who have had severe brain injury may benefit from photos or drawings that represent or capture something concrete about the value – they may prefer an audio or video summary of each value. Think about how the exercise can be kept meaningful, accessible, interesting and fun for the client – some people may prefer a pen-and-paper approach, whereas others may engage better with use of technology such as computers or tablets.

In ACT, the term "committed action" may be used over goal-orientated language. Rehabilitation is hard – exercises often bring up a lot of strong feelings – anger, hopelessness, frustration, anxiety and pain (physical and emotional) are common. This can be exacerbated by a narrow focus (often reinforced by professionals) on SMART goals (goals designed to be specific, measurable, attainable, relevant, time-based); while these can be helpful in creating focus, it can mean that rehabilitation can become centred around outcomes set by professionals (e.g. "by the first of the month, the goal is for Jim to transfer from bed to chair without assistance and to be reliably orientated to time and place"). Understandably, the person might feel these goals are not linked in any meaningful way to what they want out of rehabilitation. Incorporating values into those discussions – and explicitly connecting values with goals – supports the person to connect with the goals in a more emotional way: "Jim, you said that being independent is the most important thing to you. In order to one day be able to live in your own home, we need to practise getting out of bed, so that you can do this yourself. We know this is hard, but shall we give it a try?"

Values can also be helpful in supporting motivation and engagement with other rehabilitation tasks. Severe brain injury commonly involves problems with executive functioning, the higher-level cognitive skills that facilitate planning, self-monitoring and goal maintenance. Problems with rigidity of thought, initiation and disinhibition can make behavioural change and work towards psychological flexibility difficult. WC worked with Pete, a man who had experienced a severe brain injury several years before – he made a good physical recovery, but struggled with the functional implications of disinhib-ition and impulsivity. He found it difficult to step back and think flexibly about situations, often reacting in an angry or emotional way. This caused lots of problems in his relationship with his wife. He found it hard to remember to use the typical "stop and think" type of rehabilitation strategies (e.g. Winson et al., 2017).

Discussions around values helped to identify what was most important to Pete – being honest and being a good husband to his wife. Pete was supported to learn simple mindful breathing strategies to help him to "drop anchor" – aiming to slow down and "surf the urge" of his initial response to a situation. He was provided with a printed copy of a diagram that simply said "towards values" and "away from values" (based on the "choice point": Harris, 2019). This had more emotional resonance than other strategies he tried; it helped him to remember *why* he was trying to do things differently. We also iden-tified (and printed out) a list of values-based actions (e.g. *Value*: Honesty; *Action*: To talk to my support worker when I am upset or angry; *Value*: Being a good husband; *Action*: Going for a walk round the block before responding angrily). This approach also enabled a more positively framed focus on successes that captured the steps towards values Pete made through these small committed actions. Pete found that he was already doing a lot of actions linked to his values, and this helped to increase his motivation for further committed action, and was an important step towards a more psychologically flexible approach to life.

Conclusion

ACT offers new possibilities for those with moderate to severe brain injuries and shows good potential for contributing to successful neurorehabilitation outcomes. There is a small but developing body of research supporting the use of adapted ACT interventions for people with significant cognitive impairments. There is less clarity around the empirical effectiveness of these individualised, integrative approaches, but this type of work is always going to be informed by clinical innovation as much as empirical evidence. This is particularly pertinent for those who are unable to engage in traditional psy-chological therapy due to the nature of their impairments – ACT principles can guide more nuanced, individualised interventions with the individual, and can also be used to support a family or staff team to navigate the balance between dismissing and being overwhelmed by strong emotional responses in difficult circumstances. Although symptom reduction is not the purpose of ACT, we believe that the emphasis on psychological flexibility provides a valuable set of principles that can help to support adjustment and coping following a life-changing brain injury.

Note

1   Some real-world clinical examples have been used to illustrate the points raised in this chapter; names and identifying details have been changed and/or amalgamated with other examples to protect confidentiality.

Suggested further reading

Kangas, M., & McDonald, S. (2011). Is it time to act? The potential of acceptance and commitment therapy for psychological problems following acquired brain injury. *Neuropsychological Rehabilitation, 21(2)*, 250–276. https://doi.org/10.1080/09602011.2010.540920

Wilson, B., Dhamapurkar, S.K., & Rose, A. (2016). *Surviving brain damage after assault: From vegetative state to meaningful life.* Routledge.

References

Bai, Z., Luo, S., Zhang, L., Wu, S., & Chi, I. (2020). Acceptance and commitment therapy (ACT) to reduce depression: A systematic review and meta-analysis. *Journal of Affective Disorders, 260*, 728–737. https://doi.org/10.1016/j.jad.2019.09.040

Banks, R. (2003). Psychotherapeutic interventions for people with learning disabilities. *Psychiatry, 2*(9), 363–367. https://doi.org/10.1053/j.mppsy.2006.07.004

Beadle, E. J., Ownsworth, T., Fleming, J., & Shum, D. (2016). The impact of traumatic brain injury on self-identity. *Journal of Head Trauma Rehabilitation, 31*(2), E12–E25. https://doi.org/10.1097/HTR.0000000000000158

Bédard, M., Felteau, M., Mazmanian, D., Fedyk, K., Klein, R., Richardson, J., Parkinson, W., & Minthorn-Biggs, M.B. (2003). Pilot evaluation of a mindfulness-based intervention to improve quality of life among individuals who sustained traumatic brain injuries. *Disability and Rehabilitation, 25,* 722–731. https://doi.org/10.1080/0963828031000090489

Bombardier, C. H., Fann, J. R., Temkin, N. R., Esselman, P. C., Barber, J., & Dikmen, S. S. (2010). Rates of major depressive disorder and clinical outcomes following traumatic brain injury. *JAMA, 303*(19), 1938–1945. https://doi.org/10.1001/jama.2010.599

Boulton, N. E., Williams, J., & Jones, R. S. P. (2018). Intellectual disabilities and ACT: Feasibility of a photography-based values intervention. *Advances in Mental Health and Intellectual Disabilities, 12*(1), 11–21. https://doi.org/10.1108/AMHID-07-2017-0028

Brown, F. J., & Hooper, S. (2009). Acceptance and commitment therapy (ACT) with a learning disabled young person experiencing anxious and obsessive thoughts. *Journal of Intellectual Disabilities, 13*(3), 195–201. https://doi.org/10.1177/1744629509346173

Byrne, G., & O'Mahony, T. (2020). Acceptance and commitment therapy (ACT) for adults with intellectual disabilities and/or autism spectrum conditions (ASC): A systematic review. *Journal of Contextual Behavioral Science, 18*, 247–255. https://doi.org/10.1016/j.jcbs.2020.10.001

Chase, J. A., Ramona, H., Hayes, S. C., Ward, T., Plumb Vilardaga, J., & Follette, V. (2013). Values are not just goals: Online ACT-based values training adds to goal setting in improving undergraduate college student performance. *Journal of Contextual Behavioural Science, 2*(3–4), 79–84. https://doi.org/10.1016/j.jcbs.2013.08.002

Ciurli, P., Formisano, R., Bivona, U., Cantagallo, A., Angelelli, P., Caplan, B., & Bogner, J. (2011). Neuropsychiatric disorders in persons with severe traumatic brain injury: Prevalence, phenomenology, and relationship with demographic, clinical, and functional features. *Journal of Head Trauma Rehabilitation, 26*(2), 116–126. https://doi.org/10.1097/HTR.0b013e3181dedd0e

Doering, B., & Exner, C. (2011). Combining neuropsychological and cognitive-behavioral approaches for treating psychological sequelae of acquired brain injury. *Current Opinion in Psychiatry, 24*(2), 156–161. https://doi.org/10.1097/yco.0b013e328343804e

Gallagher, M., McLeod, H. J., & McMillan, T. M. (2016). A systematic review of recommended modifications of CBT for people with cognitive impairments following brain injury. *Neuropsychological Rehabilitation, 29*(1), 1–21. https://doi.org/10.1080/09602011.2016.1258367

Gloster, A. T., Walder, N., Levin, M. E., Twohig, M. P., & Karekla, M. (2020). The empirical status of acceptance and commitment therapy: A review of meta-analyses. *Journal of Contextual Behavioral Science, 18*, 181–192. https://doi.org/10.1016/j.jcbs.2020.09.009

Graham, C. D., Gouick, J., Krahé, C., & Gillanders, D. (2016). A systematic review of the use of acceptance and commitment therapy (ACT) in chronic disease and long-term conditions. *Clinical Psychology Review, 46*, 46–58. https://doi.org/10.1016/j.cpr.2016.04.009

Harris, R. (2019). *ACT made simple. An easy-to-read primer on acceptance and commitment therapy* (2nd ed.). New Harbringer.

Harris, R. (2020). *Values cards instructions.* www.actmindfully.com.au/values-cards-instructions/

Hayes, S. C., Barnes-Holmes, D., & Roche, B. (2001). *Relational frame theory: A post-Skinnerian account of human language and cognition.* Kluwer Academic/Plenum.

Hayes, S. C., Strosahl, K. D., & Wilson, K. G. (2012). *Acceptance and commitment therapy* (2nd ed.). Guilford Press.

Jorge, R. E., Acion, L., Starkstein, S. E., & Magnotta, V. (2007). Hippocampal volume and mood disorders after traumatic brain injury. *Biological Psychiatry, 62*(4), 332–338. https://doi.org/10.1016/j.biopsych.2006.07.024

Kangas, M., & McDonald, S. (2011). Is it time to act? The potential of acceptance and commitment therapy for psychological problems following acquired brain injury. *Neuropsychological Rehabilitation, 21*(2), 250–276. https://doi.org/10.1080/09602011.2010.540920

Lakoff, G., & Johnson, M. (1999). *Philosophy in the flesh: The embodied mind and its challenge to western thought.* Basic Books.

Lippert-Grüner, M., Kuchta, J., Hellmich, M., & Klug, N. (2006). Neruobehavioural deficits after severe traumatic brain injury (TBI). *Brain Injury, 20*(6), 569–574. https://doi.org/10.1080/02699050600664467

Locke, E. A., & Latham, G. P. (1990). *A theory of goal setting and task performance.* Prentice Hall.

Miller, W. R., C'de Baca, J., Matthews, D. B., & Wilbourne, P. L. (2001). Personal values card sort. University of New Mexico. https://motivationalinterviewing.org/sites/default/files/valuescardsort_0.pdf

Morgan, J. E., & Ricker, J. H. (2008). *Textbook of clinical neuropsychology*. Taylor & Francis.

Morton, M. V., & Wehman, P. (1995). Psychosocial and emotional sequelae of individuals with traumatic brain injury: A literature review and recommendations. *Brain Injury, 9*(1), 81–92. https://doi.org/10.3109/02699059509004574

Newby, G., Coetzer, R., Daisley, A., & Weatherhead, S. (2013). *Practical neuropsychological rehabilitation in acquired brain injury: A guide for working clinicians*. Karnac Books.

Oliver, M. A. (2020). The development and initial evaluation of the Psychological Flexibility Questionnaire-Accessible (PFQ-Ax). [Conference paper.] UK and Republic of Ireland ACT and Contextual Behavioural Science 4th Conference. www.researchgate.net/publication/349604676_The_development_and_initial_evaluation_of_the_Psychological_Flexibility_Questionnaire_-Accessible_PFQ-Ax

Oliver, M. A., Selman, M., Brice, S., & Alegbo, R. (2019). Two cases of acceptance and commitment therapy leading to rapid psychological improvement in people with intellectual disabilities. *Advances in Mental Health and Intellectual Disabilities, 13*(6), 257–267. https://doi.org/10.1108/AMHID-04-2019-0012

Pankey, J., & Hayes, S. C. (2003). Acceptance and commitment therapy for psychosis. *International Journal of Psychology and Psychological Therapy, 3*, 311–328.

Ponsford, J., Draper, K., & Schönberger, M. (2008). Functional outcome 10 years after traumatic brain injury: Its relationship with demographic, injury severity, and cognitive and emotional status. *Journal of the International Neuropsychological Society, 14*(2), 233–242. https://doi.org/10.1017/S1355617708080272

Rabinowitz, A. R., & Levin, H. S. (2014). Cognitive sequelae of traumatic brain injury. *Psychiatric Clinics of North America, 37*(1), 1–11. https://doi.org/10.1016/j.psc.2013.11.004

Roemer, L., Orsillo, S. M., & Salters-Pedneault, K. (2008). Efficacy of an acceptance-based behavior therapy for generalized anxiety disorder: Evaluation in a randomized controlled trial. *Journal of Consulting and Clinical Psychology, 76*(6), 1083–1089. https://doi.org/10.1037/a0012720

Ruttan, L., Martin, K., Liu, A., Colella, B., & Green, R. E. (2008). Long-term cognitive outcome in moderate to severe traumatic brain injury: A meta-analysis examining timed and untimed tests at 1 and 4.5 or more years after injury. *Archives of Physical Medicine and Rehabilitation, 89*(12 Suppl 2), 69–76. https://doi.org/10.1016/j.apmr.2008.07.007

Simpson, G. K., Tate, R. L., Whiting, D. L., & Cotter, R. E. (2011). Suicide prevention after traumatic brain injury: A randomized controlled trial of a program for the psychological treatment of hopelessness. *The Journal of Head Trauma Rehabilitation, 26*(4), 290–300. https://doi.org/10.1097/HTR.0b013e3182225250

Soo, C. A., Tate, R. L., & Lane-Brown, A. T. (2011). A systematic review of acceptance and commitment therapy (ACT) for managing anxiety: Applicability for people with acquired brain injury? *Brain Impairment, 12*(1), 54–70. https://doi.org/10.1375/brim.12.1.54

Surley, L., & Dagnan, D. (2019). A review of the frequency and nature of adaptations to cognitive behavioural therapy for adults with intellectual disabilities. *Journal of Applied Research in Intellectual Disabilities, 32*(2), 219–237. https://doi.org/10.1111/jar.12534

Tagliaferri, F., Companone, C., Korsic, M., Servadei, F., & Kraus, J. (2006). A systematic review of brain injury epidemiology in Europe. *Acta Neurochirurgica, 148*(3), 255–268. https://doi.org/10.1007/s00701-005-0651-y

Törneke, N. (2010). *Learning RFT: An introduction to relational frame theory and its clinical application.* Context Press.

Van Bost, G., Van Damme, S., & Crombez, G. (2017). The role of acceptance and values in quality of life in patients with an acquired brain injury: A questionnaire study. *PeerJ, 5*, e3545. https://doi.org/10.7717/peerj.3545

Van der Horn, H. J., Spikman, J. M., Jacobs, B., & van der Naalt, J. (2013). Postconcussive complaints, anxiety, and depression related to vocational outcome in minor to severe traumatic brain injury. *Archives of Physical Medicine and Rehabilitation, 94*(5), 867–874. https://doi.org/10.1016/j.apmr.2012.11.039

Westmacott, R., & Moscovitch, M. (2003). The contribution of autobiographical significance to semantic memory. *Memory & Cognition, 31*(5), 761–774. https://doi.org/10.3758/BF03196114

Westrup, D. (2014). *Advanced acceptance and commitment therapy.* New Harbinger.

Whiting, D. L., Deane, F. P., Simpson, G. K., McLeod, H. J., & Ciarrochi, J. (2015). Cognitive and psychological flexibility after a traumatic brain injury and the implications for treatment in acceptance-based therapies: A conceptual review. *Neuropsychological Rehabilitation, 27*(2), 263–299. https://doi.org/10.1080/09602011.2015.1062115

Winson, R., Wilson, B. A., & Bateman, A. (2017). *The brain injury rehabilitation workbook.* Guilford Press.

Wong, D., McKay, A., & Hsieh, M. (2012). Can psychological interventions be adapted for people with moderate to severe traumatic brain injury? *InPsych, 34*(2), 14–15. www.psychology.org.au/publications/inpsych/2012/april/wong

Ylvisaker, M., McPherson, K., Kayes, N., & Pellett, E. (2008). Metaphoric identity mapping: Facilitating goal setting and engagement in rehabilitation after traumatic brain injury. *Neuropsychological Rehabilitation, 18*, 713–741. https://doi.org/10.1080/09602010802201832

Chapter 7

Using acceptance and commitment therapy to support people with prolonged disorders of consciousness

Alistair J. Teager and Abigail Methley

Abstract

Prolonged disorders of consciousness (PDOC) are complex conditions with high medical, nursing and care needs. The profound cognitive, behavioural, and communication changes people with PDOC experience are incredibly difficult for family members to adjust to and accept. Acceptance and commitment therapy (ACT) approaches can support people to improve their wellbeing in situations where they do not have the power to directly change the situation; this is a good fit for families whose loved one becomes acutely unwell with an uncertain but likely negative prognosis. This chapter will consider how families and staff teams can name the experiences and narratives causing them distress, identify where avoidance is leading them away from their values, and develop techniques to manage these highly emotive caregiving experiences.

Prolonged disorder of consciousness (PDOC) is a term used to describe a group of diagnoses applied to those with sudden-onset acquired brain injuries from which the patient may have no or limited awareness of themselves or their environment. The term should be used to describe any disorder of consciousness that has continued for at least 4 weeks following sudden-onset brain injury (Royal College of Physicians (RCP), 2020).

PDOC has also been referred to as a "low-awareness state" or "unresponsive wakefulness syndrome" (Laureys et al., 2010). For the purposes of consistency with the Royal College of Physicians (RCP) guidelines, this chapter will use the term "prolonged disorder of consciousness" to encapsulate any disorder of consciousness that has continued for at least 4 weeks following sudden-onset brain injury (RCP, 2020). It is now increasingly recognised that PDOC form a continuous spectrum of awareness and interaction rather than a set of distinct entities. However the following categorical terms have been defined to support assessment and treatment (RCP, 2020);

DOI: 10.4324/9781003024408-9

- *Coma* – the person is unable to respond normally to pain, light, sound; they have no normal sleep/wake cycle; they do not initiate voluntary actions – they are presumed not to be awake or aware of their surroundings.
- *Vegetative state* (VS) – eye opening and sleep/wake cycles are present, but there is no evidence of purposeful response to sensory/cognitive stimuli; there is an absence of evidence for self/environmental awareness, though there may be movement in face/body (note that this term is universally disliked and frequently misunderstood).
- *Minimally conscious state* (MCS) – the person shows inconsistent but reproducible responses and there is some degree of interaction with their surroundings.

Consciousness may also fluctuate over time so that the categorisation of VS and MCS becomes blurred (Wade, 2018). It is estimated that 5–28 people per million are in PDOC (Elvira de la Morena & Cruzado, 2013; Saoût et al., 2010), and the number of people in PDOC is increasing, due to advances in medical technology leading to more people surviving serious brain injuries and neurological damage.

Prognoses for improvement and life expectancy following PDOC are highly variable and difficult to predict, being largely dependent on a variety of factors such as age, frailty and comorbidities (RCP, 2020). Common causes of profound brain injury resulting in PDOC include trauma (e.g. through direct impact or diffuse axonal injury), vascular events (e.g. catastrophic intracerebral or subarachnoid haemorrhage, and other strokes), hypoxic or hypoperfusion injuries (e.g. due to cardiorespiratory arrest or profound hypovolaemia), infection or inflammation (e.g. encephalitis, vasculitis or meningitis) and toxic or metabolic damage (e.g. drug/alcohol poisoning or severe hypoglycaemia). See RCP (2020) for further details of common causes of PDOC.

Individuals in PDOC often have significant medical, nursing and care needs. Cognitive, behavioural and communication changes are often profound. Emotional changes may be apparent, but they are difficult to assess or treat, both psychologically and pharmacologically, due to the profound nature of the aforementioned consequences (RCP, 2005, 2020).

Alongside other multidisciplinary team (MDT) members, clinical psychologists may see individuals in PDOC across the care pathway, from critical care, through inpatient and community neurorehabilitation settings, through to nursing and family homes. This chapter will aim to describe how acceptance and commitment therapy (ACT) could be applied to support individuals in PDOC when working with their friends and family and MDTs. It links to topics outlined elsewhere in this text on supporting families, supporting healthcare staff and working in inpatient medical settings.

Applying ACT with people in PDOC

Given the profound impact that PDOC has on the individual's cognitive processes and communication ability, traditional one-to-one therapy is typically not possible. However, there are a number of ways in which ACT could be applied with individuals in PDOC. Learning about the person from family and friends could help improve the person-centredness and interpretation of assessments. Ascertaining and clarifying the individual's values via family and friends could improve the care and treatment plans. For example, a life compass or bull's-eye exercise (Harris, 2009) might help the assessors learn any key values the person lived by pre-injury, for example, relating to health and relationships. The process may also, and vitally, help inform best interests in decision making (e.g. care planning, placement, withdrawal of nutrition and hydration) as this process uses their knowledge of the individual pre-injury (Edgar et al., 2015).

Understanding of the person's likes and dislikes, for example a love of film, music or being pampered, may guide the development of social and recreational activities that the family or care team can implement for the person in PDOC. Furthermore, understanding the person's values could also be integrated into behavioural support plans by helping the MDT plan and adapt environmental, social interaction, staffing and social communication interventions. For example, some individuals may historically have wished to have frequent and regular company, whilst others may have preferred privacy; some may have expressed preferences for tactile comfort or sensuality, whereas others might have wished for personal space.

Sampson[1] was a husband and father and keen footballer, who experienced a hypoxic brain injury after suffering a cardiac arrest. Sampson was transferred to an acute neurorehabilitation ward for further assessment and rehabilitation. The psychologist met with family on a number of occasions to provide emotional support and to try and find out more about Sampson. From talking to the family, the psychologist was able to ascertain that some of Sampson's most important values were hope, resilience, physical fitness, independence, family, caring and dignity. This information was shared by the family and the psychologist in a best interests meeting[2] where the collaborative decision was made for Sampson to continue rehabilitation in a post-acute specialist neurorehabilitation unit based on his rehabilitation needs and taking into account his values.

Approaching Sampson's care in this way was consistent with ACT principles for several reasons. Identifying key values improved the person-centredness of Sampson's care, and enabled family and the MDT to feel able to take committed action to maximise his wellbeing. Conversations such as these can highlight the experiential avoidance experienced by families and MDT professionals faced with complex decisions and can provide support to acknowledge narratives and step back from any that are unworkable in current circumstances (e.g. that not providing rehabilitation at home means that families are not caring, or the person in PDOC is not valued). These conversations also promoted a continuous sense of Sampson and his personhood, despite his changed circumstances, and enabled his team to share this with the family.

The experiences of family and friends of people in PDOC

Caregivers of people in PDOC may have to make highly emotive and complex decisions regarding care in a situation with little certainty. They may be concerned both about the wellbeing of the patient but also about their own wellbeing, which can feel conflicting or make it hard to live in line with their most important values. Caring for someone in PDOC commonly requires a large commitment from carers, potentially impacting employment where many hours are spent caring or travelling to the place of treatment/rehabilitation, relocating to be closer to specialist centres, loss of ability to engage in hobbies, interests and socialising, resulting in feeling socially isolated (Chiambretto et al., 2001). The prognosis for future change in a person's condition is often uncertain but it is often likely that limited change will be made; while some people may make gains in rehabilitation that can lead to improved functional ability, many people with PDOC will experience lifelong challenges. This is often difficult for families to understand; a common trope portrayed in TV, film and media shows people suddenly "waking" from a coma or PDOC, with no apparent adverse consequences.

Families may hold overly optimistic views of recovery for fear that any other approach is "giving up" on the person. Unrealistic hope may act as a way of avoiding difficult emotions such as fear of the future. Families may be dominated by self-stories and rules about how they "should" behave and care for their loved ones. At times these may be overly critical or unreasonable, for example viewing themselves as a "failure" if their loved one does not receive "perfect" care, or if their loved one seems in pain or distressed. They may set unachievable standards, such as being present at all times over a prolonged period of time, which is not sustainable and is detrimental to both their wellbeing and sustaining their ongoing lifestyle. Life may feel inflexible and unworkable.

When a loved one is experiencing hospital care, there is a large focus on problem solving, including managing day to day (finances, childcare, finding time for prolonged hospital visits) and longer-term decisions (discharge destination when prognosis is uncertain, family ability to care for the person potentially for a prolonged period of time). Reminders of the past prior to injury are painful and family, friends, colleagues and healthcare staff may inadvertently add to distress by their reactions. This highly emotive experience may tap into previous relationships and old dynamics within families.

Families experience incredibly difficult and unexpected situations where they have to adjust to the loss of the person their loved one was and the adjustment to who they are now, at a time when they are facing uncertainty about their loved one's rehabilitation and recovery (Ames, 2020). It may have been uncertain whether their loved one would have survived, and some may have prepared for their loved one's death through weeks or months of intensive medical care. It may even be that the perceived importance of different values shifts as a result of the experiences of seeing a loved one in a PDOC.

Caregivers often experience "ambiguous loss" where the person is physically available but not available psychologically or emotionally (Boss, 1999). Many varied grief responses are normal responses to an abnormal and deeply distressing situation and should be respected as such (Kitzinger & Kitzinger, 2014). However, the chronic mourning and yearning for their loved one that are experienced in these extreme situations can sometimes be conceptualised as prolonged grief disorder (World Health Organization, 2018). The experience of this comprises feeling "stuck" in a state of mourning, bitterness over loss, wishing for their previous life, sorrow and regret and feelings of emptiness and hopelessness. People experience rumination, fixation on their loss and a sense of disconnection, isolation and loneliness around others. Intrusive and distressing images about their loved one keep people in acute mourning and can prevent them engaging in the present, forming relationships and engaging in valued and meaningful activities.

The maintaining mechanisms of this experience are all amenable to ACT intervention. Many carers will not experience clinical levels of mental health symptoms but are likely to still experience increased carer burden and distress that may benefit from less intensive interventions. A self-help ACT intervention has been explored to support carers experiencing anticipatory grief and was found to be a feasible intervention (Davis et al., 2017).

How can ACT approaches help?

Opening up

The experiences that are made room for in ACT are thoughts (including memories), actions (including behaviour and urges), sensations and emotions. Its focus in grief is on helping people make sense of their experiences, making room for difficult emotions and sensations and making a new life. It presents love and loss as two sides of the same coin; one is not possible without the presence of the other.

Many carers find they experience reactions commonly targeted in ACT: they may give up, get caught in thoughts, dwell on the past or future, try to problem solve things that cannot be solved and try to avoid things that make them feel bad. They may develop avoidant coping strategies to get by during very difficult and intense times. This may include withdrawing from friends and family due to difficult questions about prognosis, reminders about how the person was previously and people holding inaccurate views on recovery. To protect them from this carers may withdraw or experientially avoid, which then limits their involvement in valued relationships and activities.

Connecting with values and doing what matters

The ethos of ACT is not to support people to reduce their thoughts and feelings but to enable them to do things that matter in the presence of difficult experiences. ACT may support people to re-engage with their values, despite the pain caused at times. This could include making plans for the future even where prognosis is uncertain, or rejoining valued groups and activities and setting reasonable visiting times, despite fears that this looks "uncaring". This could include being a caring partner even where that care cannot be reciprocated. Developing meaningful new routines and new relationships which are honouring of the person in PDOC and carers' pre-injury selves can be very beneficial for carer wellbeing (Soeterik et al., 2018). These include continued physical presence, contributing to skill acquisition and becoming experts in their loved one's care, including delivering, managing and coordinating their care (Soeterik et al., 2018).

ACT informed questions may still be of use where one member of the couple cannot respond, by changing people's attitudes towards the person with PDOC and empowering them within their situation. Identifying their values within the relationship can lead to questions such as: How do you want to be towards them? How do you want to act in your dealings with them? What sort of person do you want to be with them? What sort of strengths and qualities do you want to develop? (Harris, 2019).

Cognitive defusion

Defusion techniques help the person to notice their thoughts and step back from them, creating a sense of distance to enable new understandings and choices about actions. Defusion may enable them to name their thoughts and fears (e.g. that leaving the bedside means their loved one will be unsafe) and promote better and more helpful discussions with healthcare professionals, in turn addressing any conflict. Families may feel they need "permission" to regain valued activities and return to committed action without feeling selfish or uncaring (e.g. doing pleasurable, relaxing or leisure activities whilst their loved one remains in hospital) and defusion can enable this self-compassion.

ACT also fits well with systemic approaches commonly used within rehabilitation which support families to see their strengths and resilience. As in narrative therapy, the aim is to help people notice their "narrative" about themselves, loved ones and past events and develop a more strengths-based, less critical narrative.

Working with staff

Staff teams for people with PDOC and their families are multidisciplinary, including nurses, healthcare assistants, speech and language therapists, occupational therapists, physiotherapists, psychologists, rehabilitation consultants, dieticians and chaplains. Healthcare professionals may lack opportunities to train in working with people with PDOC and have their first experiences as newly qualified professionals with limited support and specialist knowledge. Working with this clinical group may tap into values about clinical skill and expertise, seeing improvement, supporting others and teamwork. Conversely, challenges to values may include ethics around treatment decision making, challenges to professional identity where improvement was not possible despite clinical skill and difficulties supporting families in distress (Logeswaran et al., 2018).

ACT may be beneficial in supporting staff to notice narratives regarding challenging-to-manage or agitated behaviours both with patients (e.g. pulling at feeding tubes, writhing in beds) and families who want the best for their loved ones in emotive circumstances. It may also help them reflect on their own distress at seeing people with these severe care needs and any perceptions about the rewarding and at times disheartening role of specialist rehabilitation.

Conclusion

Supporting people with PDOC presents challenges for both families and staff. PDOC are life changing and ACT principles can be applied to help maintain person-centredness of care, to help families and friends engage in difficult discussions, develop skills in living a life in line with their values in the face of distressing circumstances and support staff in coping with the emotional and ethical dilemmas that may arise.

Notes

1 Some real-world clinical examples have been used to illustrate the points raised in this chapter; names and identifying details have been changed and/or amalgamated with other examples to protect confidentiality.
2 In the UK, a best interests meeting may be needed where an adult (16+) lacks mental capacity to make a significant decision for themselves (as determined under the Mental Capacity Act, 2005). This meeting brings together key stakeholders to make the decision on the person's behalf.

Suggested further reading

Coma and Disorders of Consciousness Research Centre Training. (2020). *Introducing PDoC care*. CDOC. https://cdoctraining.org.uk/caring-for-pdoc-patients/

Royal College of Physicians. (2020). Prolonged disorders of consciousness following sudden onset brain injury: National clinical guidelines. www.rcplondon.ac.uk/guidelines-policy/prolonged-disorders-consciousness-following-sudden-onset-brain-injury-national-clinical-guidelines

University of Oxford. (2019). Family experiences of vegetative and minimally conscious states. Healthtalk.org. https://healthtalk.org/family-experiences-vegetative-and-minimally-conscious-states/overview

References

Ames, R. (2020). Systematic and narrative therapeutic work with families whose child has sustained a profound brain injury. In J. Jim & E. Cole (Eds.), *Psychological therapy for paediatric acquired brain injury* (pp. 122–133). Routledge.

Boss, P. G. (1999). *Ambiguous loss: Learning to live with unresolved grief*. Harvard University Press.

Chiambretto, P., Ferrario, S., & Zotti, A. M. (2001). Patients in a persistent vegetative state: Caregiver attitudes and reactions. *Acta Neurologica Scandinavica, 104*(6), 364–368. https://doi.org/10.1034/j.1600-0404.2001.00107.x

Davis, E. L., Deane, F. P., Lyons, G. C., Barclay, G. D., Bourne, J., & Connolly, V. (2017). Feasibility randomised controlled trial of a self-help acceptance and commitment therapy intervention for grief and psychological distress in carers of palliative care patients. *Journal of Health Psychology, 25*(3), 322–339. https://doi.org/10.1177/1359105317715091

Edgar, A., Kitzinger, C., & Kitzinger, J. (2015). Interpreting chronic disorders of consciousness: Medical science and family experience. *Journal of Evaluation of Clinical Practice, 21*(3), 374–379. https://doi.org/10.1111/jep.12220

Elvira de la Morena, M. J., & Cruzado, J. A. (2013). Caregivers of patients with disorders of consciousness: Coping and prolonged grief. *Acta Neurologica Scandinavica, 127*(6), 413–418. https://doi.org/10.1111/ane.12061

Harris, R. (2009). *ACT with love*. New Harbinger.

Harris, R. (2019). *ACT made simple: An easy-to-read primer on acceptance and commitment therapy* (2nd ed.). New Harbinger.

Kitzinger, C., & Kitzinger, J. (2014). Grief, anger and despair in relatives of severely brain injured patients: Responding without pathologising. *Clinical Rehabilitation, 28*(7), 627–631. https://doi.org/10.1177/0269215514527844

Laureys, S., Celesia, G. G., Cohadon, F., Lavrijsen, J., León-Carrión, J., & Dolce, G. (2010). Unresponsive wakefulness syndrome: A new name for the vegetative state or apallic syndrome. *BMC Medicine, 8*, 68. https://doi.org/10.1186/1741-7015-8-68

Logeswaran, S., Papps, B., & Turner-Stokes, L. (2018). Staff experiences of working with patients with prolonged disorders of consciousness: A focus group analysis. *International Journal of Therapy and Rehabilitation, 25*(11), 602–612. https://doi.org/10.12968/ijtr.2018.25.11.602

Royal College of Physicians (RCP). (2005). *Use of antidepressant medication in adults undergoing recovery and rehabilitation following acquired brain injury: National guidelines*. www.rcplondon.ac.uk/guidelines-policy/antidepressant-medication-use-adults-undergoing-recovery-and-rehabilitation-following-acquired-brain

Royal College of Physicians (RCP). (2020). *Prolonged disorders of consciousness following sudden onset brain injury: National clinical guidelines.* www.rcplondon. ac.uk/guidelines-policy/prolonged-disorders-consciousness-following-sudden-onset-brain-injury-national-clinical-guidelines

Saoût, V., Ombredane, M. P., Mouillie, J. M., Marteau, C., Mathé, J. F., & Richard, I. (2010). Patients in a permanent vegetative state or minimally conscious state in the Maine-et-Loire county of France: A cross-sectional, descriptive study. *Annals of Physical and Rehabilitation Medicine, 53*(2), 96–104. https://doi.org/10.1016/j.rehab.2010.01.002

Soeterik, S. M., Connolly, S., & Riazi, A. (2018). "Neither a wife nor a widow": An interpretative phenomenological analysis of the experiences of female family caregivers in disorders of consciousness. *Neuropsychological Rehabilitation, 28*(8), 1392–1407. https://doi.org/10.1080/09602011.2018.1529603

Wade, D. T. (2018). How often is the diagnosis of the permanent vegetative state incorrect? A review of the evidence. *European Journal of Neurology, 25*(4), 619–625. https://doi.org/10.1111/ene.13572

World Health Organization. (2018). *International classification of disorders version 11.* www.who.int/classifications/icd/en/

Chapter 8

Acceptance and commitment therapy for people experiencing seizures

Mary King

Abstract

Seizures are a common complication following brain injury. These events can lead to a diagnosis of epilepsy and/or seizures that are part of a functional neurological disorder. Seizures, whatever the underlying cause, can have pervasive and long-term implications for physical health, psychological wellbeing and functional independence. With an emphasis on "living well" rather than on symptom control, acceptance and commitment therapy (ACT) may be particularly useful for working with people with these complex conditions. Maintaining an emphasis on doing what matters and measuring therapeutic success by quality of life are particularly important in this population, given that many people do not become free of seizures.

Epilepsy is characterised by recurrent epileptic seizures (Epilepsy Foundation, 2020). Epilepsy syndromes are defined by a cluster of features (including type/ severity of seizure, age of onset, the part of the brain involved, factors that trigger seizures and brain imaging or electroencephalogram (EEG) findings). There are many different types of epilepsy, each with different aetiologies and manifestations (National Institute for Health and Care Excellence (NICE), 2012). Epileptic seizures can also be a complication of many neurological problems, including cerebral malformations, metabolic changes or infection, brain tumours or damage caused by traumatic injury or stroke (Shorvon, 2011).

The risk of experiencing epileptic seizures continues to be elevated for more than 10 years after a traumatic brain injury (Christensen et al., 2009). The magnitude of this risk depends on the severity of the injury and is further increased if the injury was penetrative, or if surgical intervention was required (Ritter et al., 2016). Overall estimates suggest that between one and five out of every ten people who have sustained a brain injury go on to experience epileptic seizures. Seizures after brain injury are thought to be caused by irregular neuronal electrical activity, potentially due to post-traumatic scarring in the brain (Englander et al., 2014; Frey, 2003).

DOI: 10.4324/9781003024408-10

Seizures can also occur as a symptom of a functional neurological disorder (FND). FND is a broad umbrella term used to describe neurological symptoms that cannot be accounted for by clearly identified physical disease or damage to the nervous system (Stone, 2013; Stone et al., 2020). Various terms and definitions have been used to describe seizures of this kind, including psychogenic non-epileptic seizures, dissociative seizures, functional seizures, pseudo seizures, non-organic seizures and non-epileptic attacks (sometimes a diagnostic label of non-epileptic attack disorder, or NEAD, is used).

For the purposes of this chapter, we have elected to use the terminology "functional neurological symptom disorder with attacks or seizures" (FNSDa), as proposed within the fifth edition of the *Diagnostic and Statistical Manual of Mental Disorders* (DSM-V; American Psychiatric Association, 2013). A full account of the historical and contextual complexities of language used in describing functional neurological symptoms is beyond the scope of this text; however we acknowledge that much of the language in this area remains ambiguous and pejorative, and use of different terms complicates research in this area. Although there is no internationally accepted terminology, we elected to use the term FNSDa within this chapter to be as contemporary and respectful as possible, as recommended by some commentators (Barron & Rotge, 2019). However, we acknowledge that no terminology is ideal.

We use the term FNSDa here to describe experiences that may appear similar to epileptic seizures; for example, involving temporary episodes of loss of control of behaviour or movement (e.g. shaking, inability to move), sensory changes (e.g. changes to vision, hearing, smell) and impaired awareness (e.g. loss of consciousness, unresponsiveness, dizziness, confusion). However, the key difference between an epileptic seizure and FNSDa is that, although many features may appear to be similar, the latter is not typically associated with changes in electrical brain activity (often measured using an EEG) that typically occur before, during or after an event (Brigo et al., 2015).

Although a variety of predisposing factors have been identified, there is a lack of consensus on the underlying mechanism by which FNSDa occur. Historically, FNSDa was considered a physical manifestation of psychological distress. More recent attempts to explain FNSDa acknowledge that the great variety in predisposing and precipitating factors means that there is unlikely to be a single causal mechanism (Brown & Reuber, 2016; Fobian & Elliott, 2019). Predisposing and precipitating factors associated with FNSDa include physical injury, trauma, alexithymia, illness exposure, attentional focus, beliefs and expectations about illness, chronic pain and avoidant coping (Benbadis, 2005; Bodde et al., 2009; Brown & Reuber, 2016; Fiszman et al., 2004; Fobian & Elliott, 2019;Marchetti et al., 2008). There is also evidence of an association between brain injury and FNSDa (Hudak et al., 2004; Lafrance et al., 2013). The causal link between brain injury and FNSDa is not well understood and is likely mediated by interactions between biological, psychological and social factors.

Differentiating FNSDa from epileptic seizures presents a significant clinical challenge which means that FNSDa is often mistaken for epilepsy at first. On average, people with FNSDa experience a 7-year delay between onset of symptoms and receiving the correct diagnosis (Reuber, 2009). Three-quarters of people with FNSDa (who do not have epileptic seizures) are treated with anti-epileptic medication during this delay, which can cause significant side effects (such as nausea, fatigue and weight gain) but does not treat the problem (Reuber et al., 2002). As many as one-third of people experiencing seizures who are investigated with video telemetry (where brain activity is monitored whilst a person is filmed) go on to be diagnosed with FNSDa and not epilepsy (Reuber, 2008).

Achieving diagnostic clarity is made even more complex by the fact that many people experience both "epileptic" and "non-epileptic" seizures. It is estimated that 20–60% of people with epilepsy also experience FNSDa (D'Alessio et al., 2006). People with FNSDa are also more likely to have epilepsy than the general population (Reuber, 2008). One study found evidence of co-existing epilepsy in 9.4% of their sample of individuals with FNSDa while another reported a finding of 36% (Benbadis et al., 2001; Reuber et al., 2003a).

Whatever the cause of a person's seizures, there can be serious implications for wellbeing, quality of life and functional independence. Many people who experience seizures struggle to find and retain employment and are not allowed to drive until they have demonstrated that they are "seizure-free" for a significant amount of time. Financial difficulties, social isolation and loss of independence are often reported (Baker, 2002; Robson et al., 2018). Many people find that their understandable attempts to manage difficult symptoms lead to increasingly restricted lives and reduced quality of life (Cope et al., 2017).

Living with the uncertainty of when and where a seizure will occur is another reason why epilepsy and/or FNSDa can be one of the most life-changing long-term consequences of a brain injury, though many people will also struggle with epileptic seizures or FNSDa without having had a brain injury or neurological condition. Both epilepsy and FNSDa have a strong relationship with mental health problems. Up to 50% of people with epilepsy have a diagnosis of a mental health problem such as depression or anxiety (Gaitatzis et al., 2004; Mensah et al., 2006; Vazquez & Devinsky, 2003). People with FNSDa are more likely to be given a diagnosis of post-traumatic stress disorder, anxiety or personality disorder, compared with both the general population and people diagnosed with epilepsy (Diprose et al., 2016).

Epileptic seizures that develop as a secondary complication after brain injury can be particularly difficult to control with medication or surgery. This increases the burden of the condition and negatively affects quality of life (Salgado & Cendes, 2009). There is a clear need for psychological support aimed at improving wellbeing and quality of life as well as managing comorbid mental health problems (Michaelis et al., 2017).

Because FNSDa is thought to be mediated by psychological factors, psychological therapy is generally the recommended treatment. The primary aim of psychological therapy is often to reduce the frequency of seizures by working on psychological factors that are thought to contribute to a person's experience of FNSDa (e.g. anxiety, stress, trauma responses). Psychological therapy also seeks to improve quality of life and reduce the burden of depression and anxiety (LaFrance et al., 2014). Although a number of different therapies have been used to treat FNSDa (including cognitive-behavioural therapy, paradoxical intention therapy and psychodynamic interpersonal therapy), currently there is limited evidence to support any specific therapeutic intervention (Howlett & Reuber, 2009; Martlew et al., 2014).

Rationale for using acceptance and commitment therapy

With a transdiagnostic emphasis on increasing psychological flexibility, acceptance and commitment therapy (ACT) could be well suited for individuals experiencing seizures, whatever the cause. Focusing on valued living rather than symptom control could be a helpful shift given that, by definition, during these events a person is not in control. Evidence suggests that only 40% of adults with FNSDa and 60–80% of adults with epilepsy become seizure-free within 5 years of diagnosis (Diprose et al., 2016). Too heavy a focus on reducing seizures could therefore be ineffective as well as disempowering. ACT does not emphasise a need to understand the aetiology of one's condition or to differentiate between symptoms associated with different diagnoses. This is useful in working with people with seizures, who may be waiting for or undergoing lengthy assessments to ascertain the underlying mechanisms behind their seizures; many of these individuals may never get clarity, especially if they are experiencing some epileptic seizures and some FNSDa. ACT offers a framework to support people to live a valued and meaningful life, in spite of the struggles and uncertainty. With the emphasis on developing a different relationship with difficult problems to allow for a more satisfying life, ACT approaches can help to improve the quality of life and wellbeing of people living with seizures.

Research investigating the utility of ACT for supporting people with FNSDa/epileptic seizures is in its infancy but has revealed some promising results. Dewhurst et al. (2015) found that individual ACT treatment for people with drug-resistant epilepsy led to significant improvements on measures of mood, quality of life, self-esteem and general functioning. Lundgren et al. (2006) found that a combination of ACT sessions (focused on acceptance, defusion, values, self as context, committed action and empowerment) and medication was more effective than medication alone at increasing quality of life and reducing the frequency/severity of epileptic seizures. Another study found that a combination of individual and group ACT sessions had a significant positive impact on quality of life and frequency/severity of seizures (Lundgren et al., 2008). Further research is needed to ascertain which, if any, ACT processes are more or less suited to people living with epilepsy.

A self-help ACT intervention for people with FNSDa was found to increase psychological flexibility and quality of life. It was also associated with a reduction in seizure frequency for many participants (Barrett-Naylor et al., 2018). Graham et al. (2017, 2018) found that participants with a variety of FNDs (including FNSDa) demonstrated improvements in mood and ability to carry out a variety of activities following a brief ACT intervention.

The practice of mindfulness (a key component of ACT-based treatments) is widely reported to help reduce stress as well as to increase psychological wellbeing and life satisfaction (Brown & Ryan, 2003; Schreiner & Malcolm, 2008). There is also specific evidence for the effectiveness of mindfulness-based interventions for increasing quality of life and reducing the frequency of seizures for people with epilepsy and FNSDa (Baslet et al., 2014; Wood et al., 2017). Developing mindfulness skills may be particularly relevant in helping to build awareness of warning signs that often occur before a seizure.

Considerations from clinical practice

The following is a brief account of ACT processes that the author has found particularly relevant when working with people with epilepsy and/or FNSDa as well as additional considerations that can be helpful.

Be present

Being present involves noticing our moment-by-moment experience, and provides the foundation for other ACT processes. There are many reasons for teaching a client the skills that enable them to be present. These include connecting with others, sustaining the focus needed to perform well on any task and increasing psychological wellbeing (Davis & Hayes, 2011).

In the context of epilepsy/FNSDa, being present also allows the opportunity for a person to increase awareness of the thoughts, feelings and bodily sensations associated with their seizures. This enables many clients to notice changes to thoughts, feelings and/or sensations that precede a seizure. Developing awareness of one's individual warning signs opens up the possibility of taking action. This might mean alerting someone that you are with, getting into a safe position and/or practising a strategy that can help to prevent a seizure or facilitate it to come and go more safely.

One such strategy is "dropping anchor" (Harris, 2019, p. 113), a technique for being present that is helpful in situations when we are struggling with a variety of difficult internal experiences. These include hypoarousal (e.g. feeling numb and exhausted), hyperarousal (e.g. feeling anxious and hypervigilant), dissociation (e.g. feeling disconnected) and overwhelming emotions.

"Dropping anchor" involves noticing your experience (e.g. thoughts, feelings, sensations), moving your body (e.g. stretching or changing the breath) and engaging with the world (e.g. noticing what you can see, hear, touch, taste and smell). FNSDa seizures can have dissociative features and strong emotional experiences can be a precipitating factor. Many people also report signs of hypo/hyperarousal and/or difficult emotions before, during and after an epileptic seizure. Stress or fatigue can also trigger seizures of any kind. There is good reason therefore to teach this skill to individuals experiencing seizures.

People experiencing seizures often feel considerable anxiety about internal bodily sensations, which might be particularly amplified in the moments before an episode. Focusing on the body and breath might therefore feel overwhelming at first. Whilst colluding with avoidance of these experiences may not be helpful in the long term, in the early stages of therapy an external anchor might be more workable. This could mean inviting someone to focus attention on their environment, for example identifying all the numbers they can see or sounds they can hear. Another option is to practise anchoring attention on an object and guiding a client to notice qualities such as its weight, texture, colour and temperature.

Being present in order to learn about one's experience can involve "checking-in" (pausing a moment to notice) at certain points throughout the day and keeping a record of the thoughts, feelings, sensations and behaviours that are observed. Through this process clients are encouraged to notice more broadly the internal experiences that they are struggling with, rather than focusing solely on the seizures. This is essential because the impact of seizures extends far beyond the events themselves, often into every area of the person's life.

Being present can also help a person to notice when their actions are being dictated by thoughts or feelings about the condition. If a person says, "I don't do X because of my seizures", we can be curious about the thoughts and feelings that mediate the relationship between seizures and behaviour. We commonly hear people describe thoughts such as "every time I do X I have a seizure" or "I can't do X because the doctor told me not to" or "I can't do X because my loved one will worry". Cognitive defusion can help people to find space to view their thoughts in different ways that might be less restrictive. Environmental factors can also trigger some kinds of seizures, so it is important to consider such information as part of an assessment process – a person recognising that certain activities seem to be linked with seizure frequency may be important information that contributes towards a diagnostic or formulation-based understanding of their difficulties.

Open up

ACT concepts suggest that we have limited control over our thoughts and feelings and that struggling with them can be futile. This understanding provides the basis for developing skills that allow us to take a step back from difficult internal experiences (e.g. thoughts, memories, sensations and feelings) – making room for them, if doing so would enable us to pursue what is important to us. Just as struggling with thoughts and feelings can lead to further suffering, so too can attempts to control seizures. Helping a person "open up" to (e.g. increase their willingness to experience), rather than struggle with, their seizures and the impact of them can help to reduce suffering and increase valued living.

To cultivate openness towards any experience, it is necessary to understand it. Finding out what a person already understands about their condition and how to manage it is important. They might have seen many healthcare professionals who have offered different and sometimes contradictory advice. A lack of understanding and access to accurate information means that stigma and pejorative narratives around FNSDa persist. Many people with FNSDa are wrongly assumed to be deliberately generating or in conscious control of their symptoms. Lengthy journeys to diagnosis can make it difficult to understand what is meant by FNSDa, and it can be hard for people to accept the diagnosis or the idea of psychologically based treatment.

Many people are initially diagnosed with epilepsy before their diagnosis is changed to FNSDa, yet continue to follow seizure response guidelines for managing epilepsy. Such guidelines, which advise that immediate emergency medical care is sought for prolonged or repeated seizures, are not appropriate for the management of FNSDa (NICE, 2012). FNSDa seizures often last longer than a few minutes and multiple seizures can happen in quick succession. However, acute medical intervention is often not of benefit and unnecessary medical interventions can lead to serious iatrogenic harm (Dworetzky et al., 2015; Reuber et al., 2003b). The confusion and uncertainty faced by people with FNSDa, their families and the professionals around them can increase anxiety, avoidance and suffering. Gaining an understanding of their seizures and how to manage them can allow for greater flexibility and the pursuit of committed action. This does not mean that we should expect to be able to answer all the questions that a person might have about their seizures. We can however support a client to seek the guidance they need from other healthcare professionals.

"Creative hopelessness" (Harris, 2019, p. 90) can support a person to assess whether the things that they are doing to try to control or avoid their unwanted internal experiences are working for them or making their life worse. This process can be applied to any unwanted internal experience, including the thoughts, feelings and sensations associated with FNSDa and epileptic seizures. By the time that most people arrive in the therapy room, they will have been living with the condition for a while. They will have probably tried various things in the hope of reducing their symptoms, such as avoiding places, situations and activities. They might have tried thinking their way out of symptoms – or they might try very hard not to think about it. They may have tried changing what they put into their bodies (e.g. via a variety of prescribed and non-prescribed substances or changing their diet). After identifying the things that a person has tried in order to control or minimise the possibility of experiencing seizures, the short- and long-term impact of each strategy can be examined, in the context of values, costs and workability.

As part of this process, it can be helpful to explore how control strategies developed. Was it a healthcare professional who advised them not to look at a computer screen for more than half an hour? Was it their employer? Was it a loved one? Was it their mind? For many people experiencing seizures, avoidance is not only supported but encouraged by the people around them. In order to take steps towards valued living, a person may benefit from developing a sense of willingness towards the experience of difficult thoughts, feelings and sensations associated with seizures. This process can helpfully involve other people in the system such as partners, families, healthcare professionals or employers. Joint sessions can also be useful when attempting to determine whether a control strategy is appropriate and serving a person well – often a plan needs to balance practical safety tips with improving a person's ability to live a valued life.

Do what matters

Knowing what matters to us and taking action that is guided by that knowledge is a core process of ACT. A person who has been living with their condition for a long time may have become increasingly guided by avoidance rather than what is important to them. There are many ways in which we can support a person to identify their values ("desired global qualities of ongoing action"; Hayes et al., 2006, p. 16). This can be hard for people experiencing seizures, who may experience difficulties with cognition as a result of brain injury, medication or psychological factors (Celik et al., 2015). A less cognitively demanding exercise that can elicit values-based conversations is to ask clients to bring in a photo or object that is important to them. Open questions can then be used to uncover values underlying their choice: "can you tell me about this photo/object?", "how did you decide which photo/object to bring?", "what does this mean to you?", "what does this photo/object show us is important to you?", "what is it like to look at this photo?"

Throughout therapy it is also important to maintain an emphasis on doing what matters. We can measure therapeutic success by the extent to which a person's quality of life can be improved. This can be difficult when a client arrives at a session reporting a reduction in frequency/severity of events. We may need to be cautious about celebrating until we have explored "what has it cost?" Some people do experience a big reduction in seizure activity, but sometimes this has happened in the context of a restricted life lived in a small and unsatisfying comfort zone. Helping a person to identify and be guided by their values is particularly important when living with long-term conditions such as epilepsy and persistent FNSDa. This focus allows people to live satisfying lives alongside the pervasive implications associated with these difficult conditions.

Conclusion

Living with seizures can have a dramatic impact on a person's life. ACT concepts can be particularly well suited for working with people with these conditions, given the individualised and transdiagnostic nature of the approach. ACT has the potential to increase the quality of life and psychological wellbeing of people living with seizures, whatever their cause.

Suggested further reading

Barr, W. B., & Morrison, C. (Eds.) (2015). *Handbook on the neuropsychology of epilepsy*. Springer. https://doi.org/10.1007/978-0-387-92826-5

Brodie, M. J., Schachter, S. C., & Kwan, P. (2012). *Fast facts: Epilepsy*. Health Press. https://doi.org/10.1159/isbn.978-1-908541-19-2

Brown, R. J., & Reuber, M. (2016). Psychological and psychiatric aspects of psychogenic nonepileptic seizures (PNES): A systematic review. *Clinical Psychology Review, 45*, 157–182. https://doi.org/10.1016/j.cpr.2016.01.003

References

American Psychiatric Association. (2013). Diagnostic and statistical manual of mental disorders (5th ed.). https://doi.org/10.1176/appi.books.9780890425596

Baker, G. A. (2002). The psychosocial burden of epilepsy. *Epilepsia, 43*, 26–30. https://doi.org/10.1046/j.1528-1157.43.s.6.12.x

Barrett-Naylor, R., Gresswell, D. M., & Dawson, D. L. (2018). The effectiveness and acceptability of a guided self-help acceptance and commitment therapy (ACT) intervention for psychogenic nonepileptic seizures. *Epilepsy & Behavior, 88*, 332–340. https://doi.org/10.1016/j.yebeh.2018.09.039

Barron, E., & Rotge, J. Y. (2019). Talking about "psychogenic nonepileptic seizure" is wrong and stigmatizing. *Seizure – European Journal of Epilepsy, 71*, 6–7. https://doi.org/10.1016/j.seizure.2019.05.021

Baslet, G., Dworetzky, B., Perez, D. L., & Oser, M. (2014). Treatment of psychogenic nonepileptic seizures. *Clinical EEG and Neuroscience, 46*(1), 54–64. https://doi.org/10.1177/1550059414557025

Benbadis, S. R. (2005). A spell in the epilepsy clinic and a history of "chronic pain" or "fibromyalgia" independently predict a diagnosis of psychogenic seizures. *Epilepsy & Behavior, 6*(2), 264–265. https://doi.org/10.1016/j.yebeh.2004.12.007

Benbadis, S., Agrawal, V., & Tatum, W. (2001). How many patients with psychogenic nonepileptic seizures also have epilepsy? *Neurology, 57*(5), 915–917. https://doi.org/10.1212/wnl.57.5.915

Bodde, N., Brooks, J., Baker, G., Boon, P., Hendriksen, J., Mulder, O., & Aldenkamp, A. (2009). Psychogenic non-epileptic seizures – Definition, etiology, treatment and prognostic issues: A critical review. *Seizure, 18*(8), 543–553. https://doi.org/10.1016/j.seizure.2009.06.006

Brigo, F., Igwe, S., Ausserer, H., Nardone, R., Tezzon, F., & Bongiovanni, L. (2015). Terminology of psychogenic nonepileptic seizures. *Epilepsia, 56*(3), e21–e25. https://doi.org/10.1111/epi.12911

Brown, R. J., & Reuber, M. (2016). Psychological and psychiatric aspects of psychogenic nonepileptic seizures (PNES): A systematic review. *Clinical Psychology Review, 45*, 157–182. https://doi.org/10.1016/j.cpr.2016.01.003

Brown, K. W., & Ryan, R. M. (2003). The benefits of being present: Mindfulness and its role in psychological well-being. *Journal of Personality and Social Psychology, 84*(4), 822–848. https://doi.org/10.1037/0022-3514.84.4.822

Celik, A. O., Kurt, P., Yener, G., Alkin, T., Oztura, I., & Baklan, B. (2015). Comparison of cognitive impairment between patients having epilepsy and psychogenic nonepileptic seizures. *Noro Psikiyatri Arsivi, 52*(2), 163–168. https://doi.org/10.5152/npa.2015.7290

Christensen, J., Pedersen, M. G., Pedersen, C. B., Sidenius, P., Olsen, J., & Vestergaard, M. (2009). Long-term risk of epilepsy after traumatic brain injury in children and young adults: A population-based cohort study. *The Lancet, 373*(9669), 1105–1110. https://doi.org/10.1016/s0140-6736(09)60214-2

Cope, S. R., Poole, N., & Agrawal, N. (2017). Treating functional non-epileptic attacks – Should we consider acceptance and commitment therapy? *Epilepsy & Behavior, 73*, 197–203. https://doi.org/10.1016/j.yebeh.2017.06.003

D'Alessio, L., Giagante, B., Oddo, S. W. W., Solís, P., Consalvo, D., & Kochen, S. (2006). Psychiatric disorders in patients with psychogenic non-epileptic seizures, with and without comorbid epilepsy. *Seizure, 15*(5), 333–339. https://doi.org/10.1016/j.seizure.2006.04.003

Davis, D. M., & Hayes, J. A. (2011). What are the benefits of mindfulness? A practice review of psychotherapy-related research. *Psychotherapy, 48*(2), 198–208. https://doi.org/10.1037/a0022062

Dewhurst, E., Novakova, B., & Reuber, M. (2015). A prospective service evaluation of acceptance and commitment therapy for patients with refractory epilepsy. *Epilepsy & Behavior, 46*, 234–241. https://doi.org/10.1016/j.yebeh.2015.01.010

Diprose, W., Sundram, F., & Menkes, D. B. (2016). Psychiatric comorbidity in psychogenic nonepileptic seizures compared with epilepsy. *Epilepsy & Behavior, 56*, 123–130. https://doi.org/10.1016/j.yebeh.2015.12.037

Dworetzky, B. A., Weisholtz, D. S., Perez, D. L., & Baslet, G. (2015). A clinically oriented perspective on psychogenic nonepileptic seizure-related emergencies. *Clinical EEG and Neuroscience, 46*(1), 1418–1422. https://doi.org/10.1177/1550059414566880

Englander, J., Cifu, D. X., & Diaz-Arrastia, R. (2014). Seizures after traumatic brain injury. *Archives of Physical Medicine and Rehabilitation, 95*(6), 1223–1224. https://doi.org/10.1016%2Fj.apmr.2013.06.002

Epilepsy Foundation. (2020). Types of epilepsy syndromes. www.epilepsy.com/learn/types-epilepsy-syndromes

Fiszman, A., Alves-Leon, S. V., Nunes, R. G., D'Andrea, I., & Figueira, I. (2004). Traumatic events and posttraumatic stress disorder in patients with psychogenic nonepileptic seizures: A critical review. *Epilepsy & Behavior, 5*(6), 818–825. https://doi.org/10.1016/j.yebeh.2004.09.002

Fobian, A., & Elliott, L. (2019). A review of functional neurological symptom disorder etiology and the integrated etiological summary model. *Journal of Psychiatry & Neuroscience*, *44*(1), 8–18. https://doi.org/10.1503/jpn.170190

Frey, L. C. (2003). Epidemiology of posttraumatic epilepsy: A critical review. *Epilepsia*, *44*, 11–17. https://doi.org/10.1046/j.1528-1157.44.s10.4.x

Gaitatzis, A., Trimble, M., & Sander, J. (2004). The psychiatric comorbidity of epilepsy. *Acta Neurologica Scandinavica*, *110*(4), 207–220. https://doi.org/10.1111/j.1600-0404.2004.00324.x

Graham, C. D., O'Hara, D. J., & Kemp, S. (2018). A case series of acceptance and commitment therapy (ACT) for reducing symptom interference in functional neurological disorders. *Clinical Psychology & Psychotherapy*, *25*(3), 489–496. https://doi.org/10.1002/cpp.2174

Graham, C. D., Stuart, S. R., O'Hara, D. J., & Kemp, S. (2017). Using acceptance and commitment therapy to improve outcomes in functional movement disorders: A case study. *Clinical Case Studies*, *16*(5), 401–416. https://doi.org/10.1177/1534650117706544

Harris, R. (2019). *ACT made simple* (2nd ed.). New Harbinger.

Hayes, S. C., Bond., F. W., Barnes-Holmes, D., & Austin, J. (2006). *Acceptance and mindfulness at work*. Guilford Press.

Howlett, S., & Reuber, M. (2009). An augmented model of brief psychodynamic interpersonal therapy for patients with nonepileptic seizures. *Psychotherapy: Theory, Research, Practice, Training*, *46*(1), 125–138. https://doi.org/10.1037/a0015138

Hudak, A. M., Trivedi, K., Harper, C. R., Booker, K., Caesar, R. R., Agostini, M., Van Ness, P. C., & Diaz-Arrastia, R. (2004). Evaluation of seizure-like episodes in survivors of moderate and severe traumatic brain injury. *Journal of Head Trauma Rehabilitation*, *19*(4), 290–295. https://doi.org/10.1097/00001199-200407000-00003

LaFrance, W., Baird, G., Barry, J., Blum, A., Frank Webb, A., & Keitner, G. (2014). Multicenter pilot treatment trial for psychogenic nonepileptic seizures. *JAMA Psychiatry*, *71*(9), 997. https://doi.org/10.1001/jamapsychiatry.2014.817

Lafrance, W., Deluca, M., Machan, J. T., & Fava, J. L. (2013). Traumatic brain injury and psychogenic nonepileptic seizures yield worse outcomes. *Epilepsia*, *54*(4), 718–725. https://doi.org/10.1111/epi.12053

Lundgren, T., Dahl, J., Melin, L., & Kies, B. (2006). Evaluation of acceptance and commitment therapy for drug refractory epilepsy: A randomized controlled trial in South Africa – A pilot study. *Epilepsia*, *47*(12), 2173–2179. https://doi.org/10.1111/j.1528-1167.2006.00892.x

Lundgren, T., Dahl, J., Yardi, N., & Melin, L. (2008). Acceptance and commitment therapy and yoga for drug-refractory epilepsy: A randomized controlled trial. *Epilepsy & Behavior*, *13*(1), 102–108. https://doi.org/10.1016/j.yebeh.2008.02.009

Marchetti, R. L., Kurcgant, D., Neto, J. G., Bismark, M. A.V., Marchetti, L. B., & Fiore, L. A. (2008). Psychiatric diagnoses of patients with psychogenic non-epileptic seizures. *Seizure*, *17*(3), 247–253. https://doi.org/10.1016/j.seizure.2007.07.006

Martlew, J., Pulman, J., & Marson, A. G. (2014). Psychological and behavioural treatments for adults with non-epileptic attack disorder. *Cochrane Database of Systematic Reviews*, *11*(2), CD006370. https://doi.org/10.1002/14651858.cd006370.pub2

Mensah, S., Beavis, J., Thapar, A., & Kerr, M. (2006). The presence and clinical implications of depression in a community population of adults with epilepsy. *Epilepsy & Behavior, 8*(1), 213–219. https://doi.org/10.1016/j.yebeh.2005.09.014

Michaelis, R., Tang, V., Wagner, J. L., Modi, A. C., LaFrance, W. C., Goldstein, L. H., Lundgren, T., & Reuber, M. (2017). Psychological treatments for people with epilepsy. *Cochrane Database of Systematic Reviews.* https://doi.org/10.1002/14651858.cd012081.pub2

National Institute for Health and Care Excellence (NICE). (2012). *Diagnosis and management of the epilepsies in adults and children.* www.nice.org.uk/guidance/cg137

Reuber, M. (2008). Psychogenic nonepileptic seizures: Answers and questions. *Epilepsy & Behavior*, 12(4), 622–635. https://doi.org/10.1016/j.yebeh.2007.11.006

Reuber, M. (2009). The etiology of psychogenic non-epileptic seizures: Toward a biopsychosocial model. *Neurologic Clinics, 27*, 909–924. https://doi.org/10.1016/j.ncl.2009.06.004

Reuber, M., Fernandez, G., Bauer, J., Helmstaedter, C., & Elger, C. E. (2002). Diagnostic delay in psychogenic nonepileptic seizures. *Neurology, 58*, 493–495. https://doi.org/10.1212/wnl.58.3.493

Reuber, M., Pukrop, R., Mitchell, A., Bauer, J., & Elger, C. (2003a). Clinical significance of recurrent psychogenic nonepileptic seizure status. *Journal of Neurology, 250*(11), 1355–1362. https://doi.org/10.1007/s00415-003-0224-z

Reuber, M., Qurishi, A., Bauer, J., Helmstaedter, C., Fernández, G., Widman, G., & Elger, C. (2003b). Are there physical risk factors for psychogenic non-epileptic seizures in patients with epilepsy? *Seizure, 12*(8), 561–567. https://doi.org/10.1016/s1059-1311(03)00064-5

Ritter, A. C., Wagner, A. K., Szaflarski, J. P., Brooks, M. M., Zafonte, R. D., Pugh, M. J. V., Fabio, A., Hammond, F. M., Dreer, L. E., Bushnik, T., Walker, W. C., Brown, A. W., Johnson-Greene, D., Shea, T., Krellman, J. W., & Rosenthal, J. A. (2016). Prognostic models for predicting posttraumatic seizures during acute hospitalization, and at 1 and 2 years following traumatic brain injury. *Epilepsia, 57*(9), 1503–1514. https://doi.org/10.1111/epi.13470

Robson, C., Myers, L., Pretoriusc, C., Lian, O. S., & Reuber, M. (2018). Health related quality of life of people with non-epileptic seizures: The role of sociodemographic characteristics and stigma. *Seizure, 55*, 93–99. https://doi.org/10.1016/j.seizure.2018.01.001

Salgado, P., & Cendes, F. (2009). The effects of epileptic seizures upon quality of life. *Journal of Epilepsy and Clinical Neurophysiology, 15*(3), 110–113. https://doi.org/10.1590/s1676-26492009000300003

Schreiner, I., & Malcolm, J. (2008). The benefits of mindfulness meditation: Changes in emotional states of depression, anxiety, and stress. *Behaviour Change, 25*(3), 156–168. https://doi.org/10.1375/bech.25.3.156

Shorvon, S. D. (2011). The causes of epilepsy: Changing concepts of etiology of epilepsy over the past 150 years. Epilepsia, 52(6), 1033–1044. https://doi.org/10.1111/j.1528-1167.2011.03051.x

Stone, J. (2013). Functional neurological symptoms. *Clinical Medicine, 13*(1), 80–83. https://doi.org/10.7861/clinmedicine

Stone, J., Burton C., & Carson A. (2020). Recognising and explaining functional neurological disorder. *British Medical Journal*, 371, 3745. https://doi.org/10.1136/bmj.m3745

Vazquez, B., & Devinsky, O. (2003). Epilepsy and anxiety. *Epilepsy & Behavior*, *4*, 20–25. https://doi.org/10.1016/j.yebeh.2003.10.005

Wood, K., Lawrence, M., Jani, B., Simpson, R., & Mercer, S. W. (2017). Mindfulness-based interventions in epilepsy: A systematic review. *BMC Neurology*, *17*(1). https://doi.org/10.1186/s12883-017-0832-3

Chapter 9

Using acceptance and commitment therapy with people with progressive neurological conditions

David T. Gillanders, Miriam Alonso Fernández
and Sarah Gillanders

Abstract

People with progressive neurological conditions face psychological challenges throughout the course of their illness. Challenges include existential threat, adjustment to an altered life course, fear of disability, as well as disability-related stigma. Activities of daily living can fluctuate with periods of relapse and remission, within an overall pattern of progressive deterioration. This can lead to a requirement to find a balance between a focus on here-and-now responding and making flexible plans for the future. A focus on the present moment and open, flexible and engaged responding can facilitate the negotiation of these challenges for the person and their significant others, making acceptance and commitment therapy (ACT) a potentially useful approach to psychological therapy. Empirical evidence for this is at an early stage but is growing and shows promise.

People with progressive neurological conditions (PNC) face a future that is at the same time uncertain and certain. The certainty is that they will continue to live with an illness that will progressively become worse over time, and that they may well die of the neurological illness or of complications caused by it. Depending on the condition, lifespan may be shortened. And yet, much is uncertain – it is impossible to predict the nature and course of the deterioration they will experience and the extent and speed at which activities of daily living, cognitive functions, fatigue, pain, impulse control and motor abilities may be affected.

In addition to changes in cognitive and motor skills, PNC can impact upon communication, social skills and sense of self. The combination of these difficulties can lead to interpersonal strain and relationship difficulties. Quality of social support and the wellbeing of caregivers can be influentia-l in moderating adjustment to a PNC (e.g. Losada et al., 2015; McCabe & O'Connor, 2012). A person's own adaptive responding – and that of their caregiver(s) – can influence their experience of their condition.

DOI: 10.4324/9781003024408-11

The neurological damage and the subsequent pattern of deterioration (and sometimes temporary remission) will differ depending on the condition. The experience of living with conditions such as multiple sclerosis (MS), Alzheimer's disease, Huntington's disease, Parkinson's disease, motor neurone disease or amyotrophic lateral sclerosis will vary greatly (see Erkkinen et al., 2018 for a useful overview). However, a shared feature of these conditions is that people living with PNC need to balance in each moment the requirement to live in the here and now versus the requirement to make plans for the future, and to adapt or let go of plans when needed. In a similar way, the person needs to learn how to ask for, accept and use help from others effectively, balanced with the need to maintain as much independence as possible. For some people living with PNC, the balance between independence and receiving help will fluctuate even within the course of a day. As the condition progresses, the requirement to shift the balance towards dependence can become more evident. Involving key stakeholders (such as partners or family members) in psychological interventions to support wellbeing, coping and adjustment can therefore be of great value.

ACT in progressive neurological conditions

The psychological burdens faced by people with PNC have led to the increased popularity of approaches centred around acceptance, willingness, values and coping. Evidence supporting the benefits of acceptance and commitment therapy (ACT) with people with PNC is growing and results are encouraging. Most of the research evidence reviewed is of case study or single-case experiment design, with a small number of feasibility or pilot studies. A recent systematic review shows that ACT-based interventions reduce fatigue, emotional distress, anxiety and depression and improve quality of life, with most of the studies undertaken with people with MS (Robinson et al., 2019). These authors further describe increases in psychological flexibility following ACT interventions. Proctor et al. (2018) further report a pilot randomised controlled trial of 27 people with MS, testing telephone-supported bibliotherapy. Although attrition was roughly a third of the sample, improvements were shown in anxiety, but not depression, quality of life or MS symptoms.

Graham et al. (2017) report a single-case experimental design series of 7 patients with muscle disorders (e.g. facioscapulohumeral muscular dystrophy, limb-girdle muscular dystrophy and vacuolar myopathy), as a proof-of-concept study. They found that four participants could be classified as responders, and three as non-responders. The responders showed improvements in depression, anxiety, quality of life and psychological flexibility. Interviews revealed that all participants found the intervention acceptable. Even amongst non-responders, there was no deterioration in function or wellbeing during the intervention.

The role of ACT processes in influencing the wellbeing of people with PNC has also been studied in cross-sectional and longitudinal studies. Acceptance has been associated with better adjustment to MS, including lower reports of distress and higher reports of positive affect (Pakenham & Fleming, 2011). Further, the impact of MS and disability stigma on wellbeing and psychological distress has been found to be mediated by cognitive fusion, supporting fusion as a useful potential target for intervention (Valvano et al., 2016). In a study of people with muscle disorders, Graham et al. (2016) showed that psychological flexibility predicted life satisfaction, anxiety and depression in cross-sectional analyses, even after controlling for illness appraisals. Furthermore, psychological flexibility was the only variable to predict life satisfaction longitudinally over 4 months, even after controlling for baseline life satisfaction, disability and illness appraisals.

Whilst not specifically focussing on PNC, there is a small literature on ACT for terminal conditions and palliative care that has relevance to this field. Serfaty et al. (2018) showed that using ACT with patients facing end of life was feasible and acceptable to them. Improvements were reported in quality of life and distress and equivalent to a talk-based control group. This does question the specific elements of ACT technology versus shared therapeutic factors.

ACT has also been used successfully in advanced cancer in two other studies (e.g. Hulbert-Williams et al., 2019a, 2019b; Rost al., 2012). Rost et al. (2012) showed that ACT improved mood and quality of life significantly better than treatment as usual, and that this improvement was mediated by reduced cognitive avoidance, consistent with ACT's mechanisms of action. Hulbert-Williams et al. (2019a) described the protocol for the BEACHeS trial (Brief Engagement and Acceptance based Coaching for Community and Hospice Settings), a modular single-case experimental design for palliative care patients. The results of this case series are not yet published in peer review, though based on conference presentation (e.g. Hulbert-Williams et al., 2019b), the results show that ACT is an acceptable intervention for end-of-life issues, with qualitative feedback suggesting that patients experienced it positively. Quantitative data were more mixed, with only one of five completers showing improvements in quality-of-life measures, two of five showing increases in psychological flexibility, two completers showing minimal changes and one completer showing a deterioration in psychological flexibility. Given that this intervention was being delivered to people with deteriorating physical health, maintenance of quality of life can be interpreted as a positive outcome.

Evidence for ACT applied to PNC is at a relatively early stage of development. Whilst the field needs more robust studies to have confidence in the findings, it does appear that the ACT approach can be helpful in adjustment to changed life conditions of people with progressive neurological diseases. Emerging qualitative research exploring the lived experience of people with neurological conditions has also highlighted the value of ACT in these settings. Farrow et al. (2020) used interpretative phenomenological analysis to explore the perspectives of people with neurological conditions who had received an ACT intervention and identified themes around how ACT supported coping and acceptance, validating people's experience rather than seeking to remove distress. Participants described a more active and engaged life after the therapy, with ACT supporting the development of a new, revised identity in relation to their illness.

Future research should focus on increasing the diversity of neurological populations studied and improving the methodological quality of studies. Such improvements include examination of the properties of useful ACT interventions, especially with those with more severe cognitive and motor impairment. Robust clinical trials with larger sample sizes, control groups and validated outcome measures are required. In addition, attrition, adherence, fidelity and acceptability data are necessary to improve future outcomes. Despite the limitations of the available evidence base, there is a clear rationale for the use of ACT-based interventions with people with PNC.

Using ACT to support people with PNC

This section of the chapter will discuss how key ACT concepts might be applied in this context. A number of simple adaptations have been found to be effective in working with people with PNC; many of the adaptations described elsewhere in this text will be of relevance here too. In particular, consider using shorter sessions, written supplements and worksheets in large text, and pictures to illustrate metaphors. Avoid giving onerous handwritten homework tasks and encourage the use of electronic diaries or alarms as reminders for exercises between sessions. Diagrams and simplified processes such as the ACT matrix (Polk et al., 2016) can make ACT more concrete and memorable for the person with PNC.

Living with awareness

ACT's focus on developing skills in present-moment awareness are relevant to achieving an effective balance between maximising independence and asking for help. In addition, the continued pragmatic emphasis in ACT on doing what is effective, what is workable, is a useful guide. Strategies such as mindfulness meditation can be effective ways to support present-moment awareness, supported by the use of recorded audio exercises.

In addition, these skills can be facilitated by altering environmental structures and routines to support awareness, and by engaging significant others in supporting such contingencies. A simple example is for a couple to arrange a regular time each day to plan the day ahead and allocate tasks depending on how both individuals are feeling, as described by Gillanders and Gillanders (2014). Awareness skills can be further developed and generalised to everyday settings by the homework task of choosing three activities of daily living to approach with a mindful quality (e.g. brushing teeth, making a sandwich, listening to a piece of music).

As activities of daily living become compromised, this training of approaching them with awareness, patience and self-kindness will be more likely to lead to effective responding. In such moments, meeting frustration and loss with the same awareness can make it more likely that the person will be able to adopt a more open, defused and flexible response to such frustrations and losses. A further important use of such awareness-based tracking is "catching" mental time travel. Whilst it is useful to make flexible plans, engage with the likely future prognosis of the condition and so on, people with PNC will report varying degrees of future-oriented worries. People can be dominated by "what ifs?", rather than living in "what is". It is important for the therapist to give space and help the client to openly talk about the future, including fears, disappointments, anger, and so on. Yet worrying, however normal, is rarely an effective strategy for living, and learning to track this automatic tendency and return to the here and now can support more deliberate, open and flexible therapeutic focus on the future.

Living with openness

Awareness building will facilitate a person's ability to track what is influencing their responding in any given moment. In-session work on workability (drawing on ideas around creative hopelessness, as discussed by Harris, 2019) can support the person to begin to let go of ineffective responding, by tracking the experienced consequences of avoidance, fusion and attachment to historical or future self-narratives. Such in-session work needs to also build in strategies for generalisation beyond the therapy room. This can be achieved by working directly in situ in challenging situations, for example supporting difficult conversations between the person with the neurological condition and their significant others, with a patient, mindful, aware and open quality. Other examples include setting up avoided activities as opportunities for developing awareness, approaching them with openness and flexible attention, and supporting the person's in vivo approach to such situations. For example, a session spent practising how to explain their PNC and the prognosis could be a useful exercise for someone who has pulled away from talking to friends about their health.

Other examples of generalisation strategies include the myriad of explicit defusion techniques or skills that a person can use for themselves to foster open, defused awareness in challenging situations. Examples include catching one's thoughts, saying them in a funny voice, singing them aloud, visualising them and making them welcome even if they are unwanted (Harris, 2019). Therapists often find it more challenging to use these types of techniques with highly sensitive content, fearing that the client will experience them as disrespectful. Introducing them with an explicit rationale, normalising and empathising with the content of the thought and deliberately stating that these strategies are intended to undermine the influence of these powerful thoughts, and not to disrespect the client themselves, can help to reduce these therapist barriers. However, the therapist will need to gather their courage, set a purposeful intention and move beyond their own discomfort if they are to make use of these strategies. Our experience in clinical work with people in palliative care settings has shown us that these techniques can have a lasting influence on developing greater openness and more flexible responding to realistic and distressing thoughts related to death and future incapacity or need for personal care (e.g. Hulbert-Williams et al., 2019a).

Altered sense of self is also a frequently reported difficulty for people with PNC. This can be because of the disruption of imagined life plans. Realising for example that a person may not have children, or may not live to see grandchildren, can lead to a mismatch between a person's hoped-for self and current self. People also frequently take valuable sources of self-worth or identity from roles and activities that they do (e.g. I am a father, a worker, a friend, etc.). As such activities and roles become compromised by neurological illness, so the person's sense of self can become threatened.

Three broad strategies are relevant here. The first involves helping the individual to adopt a more flexible set of perspective-taking skills around rigid self-narratives through enquiries such as, "What would you say to a friend who said this to you?", "What advice would a pre-illness version of yourself give to the you that is here now?" The second strategy involves helping the individual to adapt *how* they approach activities to preserve them as much as possible (e.g. pacing, planning, chunking, goal setting, asking for specific areas of help, specific adaptations to facilitate, use of aids, etc.). Even adopting such changes can involve practising psychological flexibility, as they can trigger the underlying meaning that is being avoided, for instance, "Using that aid means I am vulnerable". The third strategy involves helping the individual to move their focus from the specific activity that is compromised on to the value or purpose that it was serving. For instance, an exploration of the functions of work might reveal that it served the values of being useful to others, and of being part of a group of like-minded people. Even if a person is no longer able to work, there may be opportunities to engage in behaviours that serve these two values.

Living with values

In the early stages of a progressive illness, engaged living can actually be enhanced. When skills and abilities are relatively intact, a life-changing illness can lead to a re-evaluation of priorities and a re-focusing of energies. With good therapeutic support, this phase can help people to identify what really matters and can serve as a beacon to guide behaviour over the longer term.

It is important to frame such conversations in terms of the specific qualities that the person would most want to bring to the different parts of their life. Keeping the conversation focused on principles, qualities and domains will help to keep the actual activities that make up these values flexible. This will help them to adapt flexibly as the condition progresses and specific activities become compromised. This is a further example of how the ACT processes overlap and are interdependent; a focus on values rather than specific behaviours can help an individual to let go of fused ideas around specific activities, which can in turn lead to a more open and flexible sense of self. This in turn can lead to generation of new ideas about how to follow values.

The couple is the context

The person with a PNC rarely carries its impact entirely alone. PNC exist within a social context. For many, relationships are the context in which PNC are experienced, in particular spousal or partner relationships (Gillanders & Gillanders, 2014). Relationships with other family members and health and social care professionals can also be affected. The importance of the spousal relationship is significant for several reasons. First and foremost, a spouse or partner is already involved in actively shaping the environment the individual with a PNC lives in in terms of systems, strategies, supports, and of course in emotional tone and patterns of relating. Having this person as an integral part of an intervention will be much more likely to lead to effective generalisation of changes and skills from the therapy room to the person's home environment.

Studies have shown that the reciprocal interaction between patient and spouse (or other significant caregiving relationship) has an important influence on both the patient and significant other's mental and physical health (Pakenham & Finlayson, 2013; Starks et al., 2010). Preliminary literature reported associations between patients' and spouses' adjustment indicators (Samios et al., 2015). In one study, acceptance and mindfulness skills shaped individual and dyadic adjustment in couples coping with MS (Pakenham & Samios, 2013). These studies suggest that the couple are often an important context for the delivery of interventions. Focusing on the interpersonal adjustment of patients and relatives, increasing their psychological flexibility, may be beneficial.

Conclusion

ACT can be a useful framework for use in working with people who have PNC. ACT requires adaptation for this population, in terms of both cognitive and motor abilities, and it can be useful to consider a more systemic or couple-based approach to this work. The field is at a relatively early stage of development and would benefit from research to validate measures with more people with cognitive and motor impairments, alongside larger and better-controlled intervention studies with good descriptions of samples. Further developments in this area could also usefully explore the focus and relative balance of ACT in the earlier stages of PNC (adaptation, maximisation of function), as well as exploring the role of ACT with people in the later stages of a PNC, to support adjustment, coping and psychological wellbeing.

Suggested further reading

Bowen, C., Yeates, G., & Palmer, S. (2010). *A relational approach to rehabilitation: Thinking about relationships after brain injury.* Karnac Books.

Erkkinen, M. G., Kim, M., & Geschwind, M. D. (2018). Clinical neurology and epidemiology of the major neurodegenerative diseases. *Cold Spring Harbor Perspectives in Biology, 10*(4), 1–44. https://doi.org/10.1101/cshperspect.a033118

Yeates, G. N., & Farrell, G. (Eds.). (2018). Neuro-disability and psychotherapy, specialist topics (vol I). *Eastern influences on neuropsychotherapy: Accepting, soothing and stilling cluttered and critical minds in neurological conditions.* Routledge.

Examples of audio exercises can be downloaded for free by members of the Association for Contextual Behavioral Science at https://contextualscience.org/david_gillanders_training_page

References

Erkkinen, M. G., Kim, M., & Geschwind, M. D. (2018). Clinical neurology and epidemiology of the major neurodegenerative diseases. *Cold Spring Harbor Perspectives in Biology, 10*(4), 1–44. https://doi.org/10.1101/cshperspect.a033118

Farrow, C., Craven-Staines, S., & Hill, G. (2020). *Service users lived experience of acceptance and commitment therapy (ACT) in adjustment to neurological conditions: An interpretative phenomenological analysis study.* Manuscript in preparation.

Gillanders, S., & Gillanders, D. (2014). An acceptance and commitment therapy intervention for a woman with secondary progressive multiple sclerosis and a history of childhood trauma. *Neurodisability & Psychotherapy, 2*, 19–40. https://doi.org/10.4324/9780429466618-3

Graham, C. D., Chalder, T., Rose, M. R., Gavriloff, D., McCracken, L. M., & Weinman, J. (2017). A pilot case series of a brief acceptance and commitment therapy (ACT)-based guided self-help intervention for improving quality of life and mood in muscle disorders. *Cognitive Behaviour Therapist, 10.* https://doi.org/10.1017/S1754470X17000022

Graham, C. D., Gouick, J., Ferreira, N., & Gillanders, D. (2016). The influence of psychological flexibility on life satisfaction and mood in muscle disorders. *Rehabilitation Psychology, 61*(2), 210–217. https://doi.org/10.1037/rep0000092

Harris, R. (2019). *ACT made simple: An easy-to-read primer on acceptance and commitment therapy* (2nd ed.). New Harbinger.

Hulbert-Williams, N. J., Norwood, S., Gillanders, D., Finucane, A., Spiller, J., Strachan, J., & Swash, B. (2019a). Brief Engagement and Acceptance Coaching for

Community and Hospice Settings (the BEACHeS study): Protocol for the development and pilot testing of an evidence-based psychological intervention to enhance wellbeing and aid transition into palliative care. *Pilot and Feasibility Studies*, *5*(1), 104. https://doi.org/10.1186/s40814-019-0488-4

Hulbert-Williams, N. J., Norwood, S., Gillanders, D., Finucane, A., Spiller, J., Strachan, J., & Swash, B. (2019b). Brief Engagement and Acceptance Coaching in Community and Hospice Settings (the BEACHeS study): Development and pilot-testing an evidence-based intervention to enhance wellbeing at transition into palliative care. Conference presentation at *The Association for Contextual Behavioural Science World Conference*, Dublin, Ireland, June, 2019.

Losada, A., Márquez-González, M., Romero-Moreno, R., Mausbach, B. T., López, J., Fernández-Fernández, V., & Nogales-González, C. (2015). Cognitive-behavioral therapy (CBT) versus acceptance and commitment therapy (ACT) for dementia family caregivers with significant depressive symptoms: Results of a randomized clinical trial. *Journal of Consulting and Clinical Psychology*, *83*(4), 760–772. https://doi.org/10.1037/ccp0000028

McCabe, M. P., & O'Connor, E. J. (2012). Why are some people with neurological illness more resilient than others? *Psychology, Health & Medicine*, *17*(1), 17–34. https://doi.org/10.1080/13548506.2011.564189

Pakenham, K. I., & Finlayson, M. (2013). Caregiving. In: M. Finlayson (Ed.), *Multiple sclerosis rehabilitation: From impairment to participation* (pp. 497–526). Taylor & Francis.

Pakenham, K. I., & Fleming, M. (2011). Relations between acceptance of multiple sclerosis and positive and negative adjustments. *Psychology & Health*, *26*(10), 1292–1309. https://doi.org/10.1080/08870446.2010.517838

Pakenham, K. I., & Samios, C. (2013). Couples coping with multiple sclerosis: A dyadic perspective on the roles of mindfulness and acceptance. *Journal of Behavioral Medicine*, *36*(4), 389–400. https://doi.org/10.1007/s10865-012-9434-0

Polk, K. L., Schoendorf, B., Webster, M., & Olaz, F. O. (2016). *The essential guide to the ACT matrix: A step by step approach to using the ACT matrix model in clinical practice*. New Harbinger.

Proctor, B. J., Moghaddam, N. G., Evangelou, N., & Das Nair, R. (2018). Telephone-supported acceptance and commitment bibliotherapy for people with multiple sclerosis and psychological distress: A pilot randomised controlled trial. *Journal of Contextual Behavioral Science*, *9*, 103–109. https://doi.org/10.1016/j.jcbs.2018.07.006

Robinson, P. L., Russell, A., & Dysch, L. (2019). Third-wave therapies for long-term neurological conditions: A systematic review to evaluate the status and quality of evidence. *Brain Impairment*, *20*(1), 58–80. https://doi.org/10.1017/BrImp.2019.2

Rost, A. D., Wilson, K., Buchanan, E., Hildebrandt, M. J., & Mutch, D. (2012). Improving psychological adjustment among late-stage ovarian cancer patients: Examining the role of avoidance in treatment. *Cognitive and Behavioral Practice*, *19*(4), 508–517. https://doi.org/10.1016/j.cbpra.2012.01.003

Samios, C., Pakenham, K. I., & O'Brien, J. (2015). A dyadic and longitudinal investigation of adjustment in couples coping with multiple sclerosis. *Annals of Behavioral Medicine*, *49*(1), 74–83. https://doi.org/10.1007/s12160-014-9633-8

Serfaty, M., Armstrong, M., Vickerstaff, V., Davis, S., Gola, A., McNamee, P., & Low, J. T. S. (2018). Acceptance and commitment therapy for adults with advanced cancer

(CanACT): A feasibility randomised controlled trial. *Psycho-Oncology*, *28*(3), 488–496. https://doi.org/10.1002/pon.4960

Starks, H., Morris, M. A., Yorkston, K. M., Gray, R. F., & Johnson, K. L. (2010) Being in-or out-of-sync: couples' adaptation to change in multiple sclerosis. *Disability & Rehabilitation*, *32*(3), 196–206. https://doi.org/10.3109/09638280903071826

Valvano, A., Floyd, R. M., Penwell-Waines, L., Stepleman, L., Lewis, K., & House, A. (2016). The relationship between cognitive fusion, stigma, and well-being in people with multiple sclerosis. *Journal of Contextual Behavioral Science*, *5*(4), 266–270. https://doi.org/10.1016/j.jcbs.2016.07.003

Chapter 10

One size fits all?

Racial and cultural considerations around using acceptance and commitment therapy with people who have experienced brain injury

Rosco Kasujja, Ndidi Boakye, Nadine Mirza and Will Curvis

Abstract

Acceptance and commitment therapy (ACT) approaches may play a useful role in supporting people following brain injury. However, these approaches may not be appropriate for all – geographical, racial, ethnic and cultural barriers and disparities in accessing rehabilitation and treatment exist across the world. This chapter has been written by professionals working in the UK and Uganda; the authors will discuss pertinent issues in their countries to highlight the breadth of the challenges faced in terms of access to and availability of services supporting people following brain injury. This chapter will consider some of the potential challenges of applying ACT principles, considering issues of culture, language, spirituality and religion at institutional and individual levels. We will discuss the importance of working in a flexible and culturally sensitive way, alongside culturally competent peers within communities.

Acceptance and commitment therapy (ACT) was developed to incorporate acceptance and mindfulness strategies with values-based approaches to behavioural change, to increase psychological flexibility. Along with the corresponding theories of human behaviour – relational frame theory (RFT) and functional contextualism (FC) – upon which it was developed, ACT was created in the USA. Although mindfulness principles and techniques have their origins in Buddhist traditions and Eastern spirituality has exerted some influence on psychological therapy in the introduction of "third-wave" cognitive and behavioural therapies (Hook et al., 2017), ACT is undeniably a branch of therapy developed within a Western culture, largely used with English-speaking populations in high-income countries. Most of the available textbooks, treatment protocols and published research around ACT are aimed at English-speaking populations from Western countries. And yet, brain injury is universal. How can we ensure that we are meeting the needs of the many groups of people who do not fit this niche demographic?

DOI: 10.4324/9781003024408-12

For brevity within this chapter, we will make use of the term "minority groups" when discussing practice in the UK. We are aware that any term of this sort can be highly reductionist and othering; the word "minority" can be used to reflect a white-centric world and language, that is, assuming White is the norm against which everything else is measured – this is not our intent. When talking about race, ethnicity and culture in this chapter and using terms such as "minority groups" to describe the UK context, we refer to the powerful social factors that lead to people experiencing different levels of racialised experiences and privileges. The phrase also lacks meaning when referring to countries where people who are Black or Brown are not the "minority" (such as Uganda). Social prejudice and systematic racism and oppression are often unrecognised; when grouping people into a "minority" category, we lose the nuance and the complexity, as well as the individual and the context of their ethnic group.

However, our aim for this chapter is to shine a light on issues around racial, ethnic and cultural diversity in terms of the applicability of ACT to people with brain injuries. It is difficult to do this without referring to "White" and "minority" groups in some "othering" way, and we fully appreciate that this terminology is inadequate. Within this chapter, we seek to highlight the importance of a culturally sensitive approach to clinical work. When reading this chapter, we ask that you remember that the terminology we use is a short-hand; take care not to conflate all issues around race, ethnicity and culture. We do not propose this chapter as the final word on the matter; we hope it will spark ideas and conversations about how anti-racist and culturally appropriate services can support vulnerable people from across societies.

ACT and brain injury

Working with minority groups in the UK

Racial disparities exist across healthcare systems, across the world – these challenges are not unique to access to neurorehabilitation services, but these disparities have been associated with poorer rehabilitation outcomes and poorer quality of life following brain injury (Uomoto & Wong, 2015). We cannot separate the incidence of brain injury from the cultural, social and economic context from which it occurs; although frequency of causes of brain injuries is largely dependent on the social demographics of the area or country within which the research is conducted, research consistently indicates socioeconomic, racial and ethnic disparities in functional outcomes, marital stability, emotional/neuro-behavioural complications and quality of life following brain injury (e.g. Arango-Lasprilla et al., 2007; Gary et al., 2009).

ACT-based interventions can play a useful role in supporting adjustment, wellbeing and rehabilitation following brain injury (e.g., Soo et al., 2011), as outlined elsewhere in this text. However in the UK, people from minority groups are also underrepresented in referrals to mental health and psychology services (Beck et al., 2019). There is also a lack of representation in professional roles, with only 9.6% of qualified clinical psychologists in England and Wales being from British ethnic-minority groups (Office of National Statistics, 2018). Therefore, more needs to be done to ensure services achieve equal access and outcome equity for all. This includes developing an inclusive, highly skilled workforce, and ensuring that psychological interventions such as ACT are delivered in a culturally sensitive manner.

Working with people in Uganda

Uganda has historically been classified as a low-income country; although recent investments have seen an increase in capital development and gross domestic product, many people still experience significant poverty. Over half the children in Uganda experience multidimensional deprivations that lead to low standards of living (UNICEF, 2019). As noted above, brain injury happens within a social context; therefore it is important to note that the incidence of traumatic brain injury (TBI) in sub-Saharan Africa is much higher than the global incidence (150–170/100,000, compared to 106/100,000; Hyder et al., 2007), and the incidence of stroke in Africa has increased over the last two decades (Owolabi et al., 2015). Although the vast majority of people who experience brain injuries live in low- and middle-income countries, most of the research into acute treatment and rehabilitation, as well as the clinical resources and prevention initiatives, is found in high-income countries (Feigin et al., 2009; Johnston et al., 2009; Strong et al., 2007). Infectious diseases are often priorities in low-income countries, reducing the available resources for brain injury prevention and rehabilitation (Owolabi et al., 2015), although many infectious diseases such as malaria and AIDS commonly lead to neuropsychological impairment.

Data on the severity and impact of brain injury in Uganda are scarce, though there have been recent efforts to improve this picture (e.g. the Kampala internet-based Traumatic Brain Injury Registry (KiTBIR; Mehmood et al., 2018). Increases in the commuting population within city centres is thought to be responsible for the rise in TBIs caused by road traffic accidents (Dewan et al., 2019; Mehmood et al., 2018). The burden of strokes and other acquired brain injuries is thought to be exacerbated by poor control of risk factors and poor knowledge regarding symptoms; combined with long distances between hospitals and people's homes and poor transport options and congestion, getting to hospital in a timely manner can be difficult. This can lead to higher mortality rates and greater severity of symptoms. Due to the high costs involved in seeking treatment, many people with milder problems may not seek medical advice (Owolabi et al., 2015).

Access to neurorehabilitation following brain injury is also often limited in Uganda (Kamwesiga et al., 2018). Current treatments available in Uganda for people with brain injuries are mainly pharmacological (Bédard et al., 2012), with little provision for neurorehabilitation services, despite the physical, cognitive and psychological consequences (Bangirana et al., 2019). Kamwesiga et al. (2018) discuss how transport challenges and lack of resources (within the family and at the hospitals) can impede access to rehabilitation, alongside a potential lack of recognition of the value of rehabilitation – people who do jobs requiring physical strength and fine-motor abilities (which are more common in low-income countries) may focus on physical recovery and be less aware of or place less emphasis on cognitive or emotional difficulties.

In regard to cultural considerations for applying ACT as a treatment for individuals with brain injuries, it should be noted that psychotherapeutic services are rarely available to individuals with brain injury in Uganda. There are few professionals in Uganda using ACT in their practice. ACT has received wide coverage throughout the world since it was developed; however, it has only gained some popularity in Uganda in the last decade. There is no published literature available related to the use of ACT in a Ugandan context; this is not uncommon as research on evidence about the effectiveness of interventions is generally rare in low- and middle-income countries, although much needed (Rowe et al., 2005).

So, generally speaking, ACT is new in Uganda, hence careful considerations have to be taken before applying ACT principles. Very few specialists have had the training to be able to apply it to individuals with brain injury. There is a great need to evaluate and adapt ACT to the Ugandan setting to ensure the approach is valid and appropriate for this population. Stewart et al. (2017) report on the work of an international non-governmental organisation in Sierra Leone, highlighting the potential value that ACT might offer for building capacity for mental health in low-resource settings.

Language and cultural considerations

Issues of historical and systematic racism

Structural racism is systematic and often institutionalised. A full discussion of historical and systemic racism is beyond the scope of this text. However, awareness of racial and ethnic disparities in the context of neurorehabilitation care should alert researchers, healthcare organisations, policy makers and clinicians that disparities in other cultural groups may be suspected (Uomoto & Wong, 2015). Who is represented in neurorehabilitation services – and who is not?

People from minority groups in the UK accessing services in medical or rehabilitation settings may be more apprehensive or anxious. The consequences of historical examples of institutional racism in healthcare settings reverberate through generations (e.g. the Tuskegee experiment conducted in Alabama between 1932 and 1972, an observational study where

300 Black men with syphilis were not told about their condition or given treatment, even after penicillin became widely available). Even in the 21st century, race continues to be inseparable from healthcare; in 2020, Black people in the UK were more than four times as likely as White people to be detained under the Mental Health Act (UK Government, 2021). In terms of COVID-19, people from minority groups in the UK – particularly males of Black African, Black Caribbean and Bangladeshi ethnic backgrounds – had the highest rates of mortality (Office of National Statistics, 2020). In countries like Uganda, racism and colonialism continue to be connected to resource provision and access to services; there is limited capacity to develop and fund initiatives and research into homegrown interventions, tailored to the need of the population.

These problems are multi-faceted and longstanding, but distrust of health and mental health services (due to discrimination), lack of consistency in diagnosis, exposure to deprivation and reduced social support continue to affect the health and wellbeing of people from minority groups in the UK (Godlee, 2020). Funding for healthcare and specialist rehabilitation services is not equitable across the world, with low- and middle-income countries having significantly fewer resources to apply to these sectors. Professionals and therapists have a responsibility to be aware of this context and a duty to make services as safe and accessible as possible. In order to deliver culturally responsive ACT interventions, clinicians must first have an awareness of discrimination, bias, their own stereotypes and the effects of overt and structural racism (Sue & Sue, 2003).

Issues around cultural beliefs and biases

Psychological therapies always need to be adapted to meet the individual's needs and circumstances (Beck et al., 2019; Nagayama et al., 2019). Alongside racial, cultural and ethnic background, a person's religious and spiritual identity, gender norms and individual life experiences should be considered (Hook et al., 2017). Within ACT approaches, it is key to consider values at both individual and community levels, as well as cultural differences regarding components of ACT (such as mindfulness principles).

However, when thinking about how this works in the UK, using ACT (or indeed any psychological intervention) with someone from a minority group requires careful consideration – especially as these interventions are delivered by majority White healthcare professionals, within systems where systemic and organisational discrimination occurs. Cultural differences may lead to misunderstandings between the person and the professional. For example, the rehabilitation setting can mimic acute care hospital settings; this setting may be seen as providing "traditional" medical treatment, as understandings of roles within this context are culturally and socially created (e.g. doctors and nurses care for patients, whereas patients take a passive role receiving treatment and waiting for results). This view may be interpreted by professionals as "poor engagement" in rehabilitation or therapy, or evidence of a lack of "psychological mindedness", resulting in psychological intervention being withdrawn or not offered.

Cultural context also drives a person's priorities within therapy and rehabilitation, based on their beliefs or attitudes. For example, a higher proportion of people in low- and middle-income countries have jobs that require physical strength and fine-motor abilities – combined with financial pressures, this may lead to them prioritising physical aspects of rehabilitation and less focus on the cognitive or psychological sequalae of brain injury. This is especially pertinent for services that are not free at point of access or require time-consuming and costly travel; services can become hard or impossible for many people to reach. This is a particular challenge in Uganda, where many communities live a long way from the hospitals where rehabilitation services are provided.

After brain injury, it is common to see stigma, misconceptions and misattributions around behaviours which challenge staff (e.g. poor engagement, verbal aggression or physical violence). McClure (2011) suggested that these misattributions are reflective of the "invisible" nature of many disabilities caused by brain injury, and the tendency to make inappropriate comparisons about what constitutes normal or typical behaviour, as opposed to examining changes within a person before and after an injury. To our knowledge, no research has explored how stigma or misunderstanding from a brain injury perspective might intersect with the enduring negative stereotypes that exist around violent or "anti-social" behaviour around Black and marginalised groups (Alexander, 2012; Peralta, 2010; Peralta et al., 2019). See Peralta et al. (2019) for a useful summary of the available research around the social construction of Black violence and the impact of systemic racism (particularly in the criminal justice system) on societal narratives around violence and race.

If these misunderstandings and misattributions can be overcome, ACT-based interventions could play a useful role in supporting reflection on values and improved engagement for the person needing rehabilitation, while also helping to highlight and challenge unrecognised unconscious biases that professionals can hold. ACT principles could play a useful role in supporting professionals to think about "fused" thoughts and beliefs that might be at play, and to help them reflect on the values they want to bring to how they work positively with the people under their services.

Cultural context will also heavily influence the emotional experience of brain injury. Brain injury can cause a range of visible and invisible physical and social disabilities, such as physical disfigurement, amputation, dysarthria, dysexecutive or disinhibited behaviours or decreased social cognition. Such disabilities are often misunderstood and can also make both an individual and their family feel stigmatised; perceived stigma can reduce social and community participation (Poritz et al., 2019) and affect psychological wellbeing (e.g. social anxiety; Curvis et al., 2018). The cultural aspects of stigma and shame – at both individual levels and community/society levels – will shape how a person engages with support and rehabilitation after brain injury. Simple adaptations to ACT-based approaches – such as clarifying and regularly reaffirming confidentiality policies – may support engagement.

Other considerations or adaptations from professionals may be similarly simple in theory, but are often not applied in practice. Making questionnaires or reading materials understandable or offering a choice of therapist (e.g. based on age, gender) often does not happen – even though in some communities within Uganda, offence may be caused by the idea of a younger person treating an older person. Gestures, phrases or even body language (e.g. physical contact or space) will have different meanings across different racial, ethnic and cultural groups. Many professionals feel uncomfortable or awkward about naming and discussing difference in a positive and curious way, which can lead to difficulties; however, what is perhaps even more problematic is when these differences go unnoticed and unacknowledged.

Indeed, unconscious biases often go unrecognised, even as they are employed – for example, in the explanation of ACT as a therapeutic model, the metaphors, language and stories that are drawn on come from the cultures of the majority – and may not be accessible or understandable for people from other cultures. For example, the chessboard metaphor on internal struggles and self-as-context by Harris (2019) would not be understood by many people in Uganda, particularly those in more rural areas. Every analogy or metaphor is laden with cultural baggage.

Despite the best intentions, professionals can create therapeutic spaces that are difficult for people to enter and access – either practically, or in terms of the approach, model or intervention just not being a good "fit". For example, people from some cultural groups do not readily speak about certain topics – if talking about one's own thoughts is not seen as appropriate, defusion work within ACT could be difficult. In some communities in Uganda and minority groups in the UK, people from an older generation would find it disrespectful for a therapist to ask them what they are thinking. Adaptations – such as encouraging the person to write down their thoughts rather than disclose them to the therapist – may be possible, but would need to be developed carefully and collaboratively. This kind of adaptation may be more challenging for people who have experienced brain injury.

Furthermore, it is important to be mindful that people from minority groups in countries like the UK have experienced repeated trauma of cultural loss due to policies and cultural experiences of "Whiteness" in their communities (e.g. suppression of native languages and cultural practices). Traditional applications of ACT may be seen as another example of this. The ACT therapist may wish to enter into this process with curiosity and guidance from the people they are working with about what may best support them to access

ACT. This will serve to build trust, a fundamental principle in developing rapport and essential for good therapeutic outcomes. Co-construction is key; for example, a joint training venture between Rosco Kasujja and Ross White highlighted the potential value of applying ACT principles in Uganda, showing that this could be applied in a culturally sensitive way which considered how notions of overcoming difficulties are captured in different languages used in Uganda, poems and songs (White, 2017).

Hook et al. (2017) describe the concept of cultural humility – the ability to maintain an interpersonal stance that considers the culture of the other person in a non-judgemental way. They highlight various processes of critical self-reflection, including being open to learning, being self-aware, being ego-less and facilitating supportive interactions. Continual examination of the power imbalances within therapeutic relationships, alongside broader strategies to value multiculturalism such as service evaluation, hiring practices that support inclusivity and diversity, partnerships with communities and institutional goals around education have been described as the best ways to support mutual empowerment and optimal care, centred around respect and partnership working (Foronda et al., 2015).

Issues around language

A full discussion of the intricacies around language is unfortunately beyond the scope of this chapter. But diversity in language is common, especially when working in multicultural communities found in both the UK and Uganda. This diversity has the potential to affect all aspects of any clinical psychology practice; therapy is relational, and relationships are built on language and communication (Espín, 2013). The subtle and complex meanings behind the words used by both client and therapist are a crucial component of any therapeutic intervention. Within ACT, an approach built around principles of RFT, the argument could be made that use of language is even more important – the way we talk about thoughts, feelings and experiences is a fundamental component of the approach.

As touched on earlier, many healthcare professionals are English speaking; yet English is commonly not a client's first language. Many people in the UK are bilingual. Uganda is a diverse country, made up of people from different regions and different tribes. Most Ugandans do not consider English to be their mother tongue even though it is widely used and considered the official language; yet Uganda does not have any training programme that teaches people to conduct therapy in their mother tongue. This restricts the application of ACT to interpretation and translation. When working with people who have experienced a brain injury, dialect and language variables also have a powerful effect on assessment performance (Fernández & Abe, 2017). It is critical to take this into account when doing any neuropsychological assessment or therapy. English skills learned as a second language may be more impaired when compared to the person's native language. People may be seen as more impaired than they truly are if an assessment cannot be completed in their first language. Conversely, more subtle impairments may be missed or overlooked. Appropriate normative data for neuropsychological assessment tools are often lacking. This is also broader than just language; many neuropsychological test batteries and tools were developed with Western populations in mind, and may not be valid or reliable within other populations. Even if translated versions are available, cultural validation is important (see Mirza et al., 2018).

Interpreters have commonly been used to bridge a gap when working with linguistically diverse populations. However, this can be anxiety provoking for the patient if the patient and the interpreter are from small communities, and it is possible that there may be dual relationships. This can make confidentiality and therefore trust a challenge. The therapist is advised to check with the patient and/ or their families as to how they may wish to navigate the challenge of language. The therapist should also work closely with the interpreter to ensure that both parties are appropriately trained to work together, for example, considering issues around the importance of language choice (i.e. not putting their own interpretations on what the client is trying to say), body language, seating arrangements and confidentiality. Debriefing an interpreter after a session may be useful. Guidelines for working with interpreters are available (British Psychological Society, 2017; North West London NHS Foundation Trust, 2016). As in many low- and middle-income countries, there are not always sufficient numbers of highly trained interpreters available to support mental health-related work in Uganda. ACT material should be passed on to specialists and non-specialists in a language that is easily understandable to Ugandans (trainees and clients) because most Ugandans do not consider English to be their mother tongue.

Issues around spirituality and religion

While many approaches to psychological therapy are conceptually distant from any religious influence, it is not easy to claim the same for ACT. ACT incorporates mindfulness principles, which have their roots in Buddhism (Fung, 2014). Buddhism is not a mainstream religion in either the UK or Uganda. Uganda is a strongly religious country, with most people consulting either religious or traditional healers to get services ranging from health, wealth and wisdom. Sorsdahl et al. (2009) reported that the majority of individuals presenting at mental health units in Uganda have previously visited a traditional, spiritual and faith practitioner. In the UK, many ethnic-minority communities rely heavily on religious organisations and communities for spiritual guidance and support. Clinically, this can be a barrier to psychological therapy as spirituality and psychology can often be viewed as mutually exclusive – if someone sees an approach to psychological therapy as being inconsistent with their religion, they are unlikely to engage.

Additionally, brain injury may be a challenge to a person's religion or spirituality. The person may believe they are being punished or ignored by their faith. Physical, sensory, communication or cognitive impairments may make it more difficult for people to connect with their faith. However, research suggests that, following acquired brain injury, spirituality can play an important role in the recovery process (Jones et al., 2018). By incorporating Eastern and Western religious and spiritual traditions, the inherent principles of ACT mean that it is possible to see it as a bridge between spiritual and psychological care (Nieuwsma et al., 2016).

ACT does not seek to change people's thinking; rather, people are encouraged to accept the content of their thoughts and emotions in a non-judgemental way, while making committed changes to live by the values they choose. This does not need to be centred around religion, though the person may find it connects to themes or topics from their religious or spiritual background. ACT provides a space for people to reflect on where their values come from and how the "rules for living" they have might sit with these values. Mapping ACT concepts with those promoted in the patient's spiritual/religious beliefs could be a useful way to link spiritual with psychological care (e.g. the ACT concept of living according to your values could be seen as akin to living as Jesus lived in Christianity). ACT may offer a useful set of principles that could help someone to reconnect with the religious or spiritual aspects of themselves, guided by their personal values and the values of their community.

However, careful consideration needs to be taken when integrating ACT ideas into therapy or rehabilitation, or when training service providers in this. It is important to emphasise that ACT does not aim to change someone's faith, nor is it a religion of any sort. It may be more appropriate to focus on mindfulness as a process of shifting attention, rather than conceptualising it as a more spiritual process of "meditation" – but this will depend on the individual. Any miscommunication about this might create difficulties in rehabilitation or therapy. In Uganda it would be of great importance to liaise with both traditional and faith healers first, as a form of building capacity, and second, as a way to ensure that more people are recommended to (and retained in) therapy. Conversely, in the UK, psychology services are often quite separate from religious groups or services in communities, with an emphasis on individualised work rather than community-based interventions. If we are to truly embed neuropsychology services into the communities we serve, an approach based on joint working and collaboration may be valuable.

Working alongside culturally competent peers

A community-based approach, which involves developing internal and external links with culturally competent members of the health and community system (including multi-faith services), is critical to building trust and opening a dialogue about the benefits of rehabilitation and psychological approaches such as ACT following brain injury.

In Uganda qualified mental health "experts" tend to be concentrated in urban areas – specifically Kampala, or areas surrounding the city (Shah et al., 2017). However, approximately 75% of Ugandan households are in rural areas (Uganda Bureau of Statistics, 2016). This means that there is a marked shortage of professionals available to meet the psychological needs of the large number of Ugandans living in rural settings. Training individuals from rural areas in approaches such as ACT may help to address some of this need.

Recruitment and training of peer support workers, experts by experience and lay health workers have been shown to play a useful role in increasing the delivery of psychologically based interventions in both high- and low-income countries (e.g. Ryan et al., 2019; Shahmalak et al., 2019). The concept of "task shifting" or "task sharing" (i.e. delegating tasks such as the delivery away from a small number of highly trained professionals to a larger number of people with minimum training) has been employed to increase the coverage of mental health care and to use limited resources more efficiently across communities (Shahmalak et al., 2019; Mendenhall et al., 2014). Appropriate training around brain injury, rehabilitation and approaches such as ACT would be required. Supervision and support for these workers are also vital, alongside appropriate financial recompense. However, community-based approaches such as these have the potential to be more culturally and ecologically sensitive, drawing on the strengths and resources of the community while redistributing power and expertise to a broader range of people.

It could be argued that working alongside culturally competent peers happens less in the UK – although the challenges facing services in the UK may be different, this could also be a useful way to support cultural humility and develop positive working relationships. The power and "expertise" around psychological therapy and neurorehabilitation are often held by professionals working in services. We believe that much could be learned from principles of community psychology (e.g. Levine & Perkins, 1997; Smail, 2005) in terms of how brain injury services might draw on the expertise of community-based organisations, religious groups and peer-led organisations.

Though not specific to ACT or brain injury work, two of the authors of this chapter (RK and WC) are involved with Sharing Stories, a collaborative venture promoting mental health in the UK and Uganda, based on the mutual exchange of ideas, knowledge and experience between people who work in and/or use mental health services. Sharing Stories has been involved in a diverse range of projects to support mental wellbeing in both the UK and Uganda, developing close links with partner organisations and university training communities. Through collaboration, shared learning and mutual respect, ventures such as these can offer useful insights into how professionals and the services in which they work can become more culturally sensitive and meet the needs of the populations they serve.

Conclusion

ACT is a potentially useful approach to support the wellbeing of people who have experienced brain injuries, but careful thought needs to be given to ensure that any interventions are culturally appropriate. This chapter has highlighted some considerations that might be relevant in thinking about how to ensure that the needs of all people who might need support after brain injury are met. This is by no means exhaustive; the only approach that can work is an open and curious one. Developing an inclusive, highly skilled workforce requires investment and training, to ensure that professionals (of any background and level of qualification) feel able to consider and challenge the cultural assumptions in the approaches they are using and embody a position of cultural humility.

Suggested further reading

Hook, J. N., Davis, D., Owen, J., & DeBlaere, C. (2017). *Cultural humility: Engaging diverse identities in therapy*. American Psychological Association. https://doi.org/10.1037/0000037-000

Nieuwsma, J. A., Walser, R. D., Hayes, S. C., & Tan, S.-Y. (Eds.) (2016). ACT for clergy and pastoral counselors. *Using acceptance and commitment therapy to bridge psychological and spiritual care*. Context Press.

Uomoto, M. J., & Wong, T. (2015). *Multicultural neurorehabilitation: Clinical principles for rehabilitation professionals*. Springer. https://doi.org/10.1891/9780826115287

Sharing Stories Venture – read more at www.sharingstoriesventure.com/

References

Alexander, M. (2012). *The new Jim Crow: Mass incarceration in the age of colorblindness*. The New Press.

Arango-Lasprilla, J. C., Rosenthal, M., Deluca, J., Komaroff, E., Sherer, M., Cifu, D., & Hanks, R. (2007). Traumatic brain injury and functional outcomes: Does minority status matter? *Brain Injury*, 21(7), 701–708. https://doi.org/10.1080/02699050701481597

Bangirana, P., Giordani, B., Kobusingye, O., Murungyi, L., Mock, C., John, C. C., & Idro, R. (2019). Patterns of traumatic brain injury and six-month neuropsychological outcomes in Uganda. *BMC Neurology*, 19(1). https://doi.org/10.1186/s12883-019-1246-1

Beck, A., Naz, S., Brooks, M., & Jankowska, M. (2019). *Black, Asian and minority ethnic service users positive practice guide*. BABCP. https://legacy.babcp.com/files/IAPT-BAME-PPG-2019.pdf

Bédard, M., Felteau, M., Marshall, S., Dubois, S., Gibbons, C., & Klein, R. (2012). Mindfulness-based cognitive therapy: Benefits in reducing depression following a traumatic brain injury. *Advances in Mind–Body Medicine, 26*(1), 14–20. https://doi.org/10.1097/htr.0b013e3182a615a0

British Psychological Society. (2017). *Working with interpreters: Guidelines for psychologists.* www.bps.org.uk/sites/www.bps.org.uk/files/Policy/Policy%20-%20Files/Working%20with%20interpreters%20-%20guidelines%20for%20psychologists.pdf

Curvis, W., Simpson, J., & Hampson, N. (2018). Social anxiety following traumatic brain injury: An exploration of associated factors. *Neuropsychological Rehabilitation, 28*(4), 527–547. https://doi.org/10.1080/09602011.2016.1175359

Dewan, M. C., Rattani, A., Gupta, S., Baticulon, R. E., Hung, Y.-C., Punchak, M., & Park, K. B. (2019). Estimating the global incidence of traumatic brain injury. *Journal of Neurosurgery, 130*(4), 1080–1097. https://doi.org/10.3171/2017.10.jns17352

Espín, O. M. (2013). Making love in English: Language in psychotherapy with immigrant women. *Women & Therapy, 36*(3–4), 198–218. https://doi.org/10.1080/02703149.2013.797847

Feigin, V. L., Lawes, C. M., Bennett, D. A., Barker-Collo, S. L., & Parag, V. (2009). Worldwide stroke incidence and early case fatality reported in 56 population-based studies: A systematic review. *The Lancet Neurology, 8*(4), 355–369. https://doi.org/10.1016/s1474-4422(09)70025-0

Fernández, A. L., & Abe, J. (2017). Bias in cross-cultural neuropsychological testing: Problems and possible solutions. *Culture and Brain, 6*(1), 1–35. https://doi.org/10.1007/s40167-017-0050-2

Foronda, C., Baptiste, D.-L., Reinholdt, M. M., & Ousman, K. (2015). Cultural humility. *Journal of Transcultural Nursing, 27*(3), 210–217. https://doi.org/10.1177/1043659615592677

Fung, K. (2014). Acceptance and commitment therapy: Western adoption of Buddhist tenets? *Psychology & Counselling, 52*(4), 561–576. https://doi.org/10.1177%2F1363461514537544

Gary, K. W., Arango-Lasprilla, J. C., & Stevens, L. F. (2009). Do racial/ethnic differences exist in post-injury outcomes after TBI? A comprehensive review of the literature. *Brain Injury, 23*(10), 775–789. https://doi.org/10.1080/02699050903200563

Godlee, F. (2020). Racism: The other pandemic. *BMJ*, m2303. https://doi.org/10.1136/bmj.m2303

Harris, R. (2019). *ACT made simple* (2nd ed.). New Harbinger.

Hook, J. N., Davis, D., Owen, J., & DeBlaere, C. (2017). *Cultural humility: Engaging diverse identities in therapy.* American Psychological Association. https://doi.org/10.1037/0000037-000

Hyder, A. A., Wunderlich, C. A., Puvanachandra, P., Gururaj, G., & Kobusingye, O. C. (2007). The impact of traumatic brain injuries: A global perspective. *NeuroRehabilitation, 22*(5), 341–353. https://doi.org/10.3233/nre-2007-22502

Johnston, S. C., Mendis, S., & Mathers, C. D. (2009). Global variation in stroke burden and mortality: Estimates from monitoring, surveillance, and modelling. *The Lancet Neurology, 8*(4), 345–354. https://doi.org/10.1016/s1474-4422(09)70023-7

Jones, F. K., Pryor, J., Care-Unger, C., & Simpson, K. G. (2018). Spirituality and its relationship with positive adjustment following traumatic brain injury: A scoping review. *Brain Injury, 32*(13–14), 1612–1622. https://doi.org/10.1080/02699052.2018.1511066

Kamwesiga, J. T., Von Kock, L. K., Eriksson, G. M., & Guidetti, S. G. E. (2018). The impact of stroke on people living in central Uganda: A descriptive study. *African Journal of Disability*, 7. https://doi.org/10.4102/ajod.v7i0.438

Levine, M., & Perkins, D. V. (1997). *Principles of community psychology: Perspectives and applications* (2nd ed.). Oxford University Press.

McClure, J. (2011). The role of causal attributions in public misconceptions about brain injury. *Rehabilitation Psychology*, 56(2), 85–93. https://doi.org/10.1037/a0023354

Mehmood, A., Zia, N., Hoe, C., Kobusingye, O., Ssenyojo, H., & Hyder, A. A. (2018). Traumatic brain injury in Uganda: Exploring the use of a hospital based registry for measuring burden and outcomes. *BMC Research Notes*, 11(1). https://doi.org/10.1186/s13104-018-3419-1

Mendenhall, E., De Silva, M. J., Hanlon, C., Petersen, I., Shidhaye, R., Jordans, M., Luitel, N., Ssebunnya, J., Fekadu, A., Patel, V., Tomlinson, M., & Lund, C. (2014). Acceptability and feasibility of using non-specialist health workers to deliver mental health care: Stakeholder perceptions from the PRIME district sites in Ethiopia, India, Nepal, South Africa, and Uganda. *Social Science & Medicine*, 118, 33–42. https://doi.org/10.1016/j.socscimed.2014.07.057

Mirza, N., Panagioti, M., & Waheed, W. (2018). Cultural validation of the Addenbrooke's Cognitive Examination Version III Urdu for the British Urdu-speaking population: A qualitative assessment using cognitive interviewing. *BMJ Open*, 8(12), e021057. https://doi.org/10.1136/bmjopen-2017-021057

Nagayama, G. C., Kim-Mozeleski, J. E., Zane, N. W., Sato, H., Huang, E. R., Tuan, M., & Ibaraki, A. Y. (2019). Cultural adaptations of psychotherapy: Therapists' applications of conceptual models with Asians and Asian Americans. *Asian American Journal of Psychology*, 10(1), 68–78. https://doi.org/10.1037/aap0000122

Nieuwsma, J. A., Walser, R. D., Hayes, S. C., & Tan, S. (2016). *ACT for clergy and pastoral counselors: Using acceptance and commitment therapy to bridge psychological and spiritual care*. Context Press.

North West London NHS Foundation Trust. (2016). *An electronic resource handbook for CNWL memory services: Dementia information for Black, Asian and minority ethnic communities*. www.scie-socialcareonline.org.uk/an-electronic-resource-handbook-for-cnwl-memory-services-dementia-information-for-black-asian-and-minority-ethnic-communities/r/a11G0000009TDcfIAG

Office of National Statistics. (2018). *Ethnicity and national identity in England and Wales*. www.ons.gov.uk/peoplepopulationandcommunity/culturalidentity/ethnicity/articles/ethnicityandnationalidentityinenglandandwales/previousReleases

Office of National Statistics. (2020). *Updating ethnic contrasts in deaths involving the coronavirus (COVID-19), England and Wales: Deaths occurring 2 March to 28 July 2020*. www.ons.gov.uk/peoplepopulationandcommunity/birthsdeathsandmarriages/deaths/articles/updatingethniccontrastsindeathsinvolvingthecoronaviruscovid19englandandwales/deathsoccurring2marchto28july2020#:~:text=In%20England%20and%20Wales%2C%20males%20of%20Black%20African%2C%20Black%20Caribbean,than%20all%20other%20ethnic%20groups

Owolabi, M., Akarolo-Anthony, S., Akinyemi, R., Arnett, D., Gebregziabher, M., Jenkins, C., & Ovbiagele, B. (2015). The burden of stroke in Africa: A glance at the present and a glimpse into the future. *Cardiovascular Journal of Africa, 26*(2), S27–S38. https://doi.org/10.5830/cvja-2015-038

Peralta, R. L. (2010). Raced and gendered reactions to the deviance of drunkenness: A sociological analysis of race and gender disparities in alcohol use. *Contemporary Drug Problems, 37*(3), 381–415. https://doi.org/10.1177/009145091003700303

Peralta, R. L., Merrill, M., Chervenak Wiley, L., Rosen, N., & Bosich, P. N. (2019). Unraveling the intersecting meanings of interpersonal violence: The embodiment of gender and race in attributions and characterizations of violence. *Deviant Behavior, 41*(9), 1125–1142. https://doi.org/10.1080/01639625.2019.1596551

Poritz, J. M. P., Harik, L. M., Vos, L., Ngan, E., Leon-Novelo, L., & Sherer, M. (2019). Perceived stigma and its association with participation following traumatic brain injury. *Stigma and Health, 4*(1), 107–115. https://doi.org/10.1037/sah0000122

Rowe, K. A., de Savigny. D., Lanata, F. C., & Victora, G. C. (2005). How can we achieve and maintain high-quality performance of health workers in low-resource settings? A review. *The Lancet, 366*(9490), 1026–1035. https://doi.org/10.1016/s0140-6736(05)67028-6

Ryan, G. K., Kamuhiirwa, M., Mugisha, J., Baillie, D., Hall, C., Newman, C., & Mpango, R. (2019). Peer support for frequent users of inpatient mental health care in Uganda: Protocol of a quasi-experimental study. *BMC Psychiatry, 19*(1). https://doi.org/10.1186/s12888-019-2360-8

Shah, A., Wheeler, L., Sessions, K., Kuule, Y., Agaba, E., & Merry, S. P. (2017). Community perceptions of mental illness in rural Uganda: An analysis of existing challenges facing the Bwindi Mental Health Programme. *African Journal of Primary Health Care & Family Medicine, 9*(1). https://doi.org/10.4102/phcfm.v9i1.1404

Shahmalak, U., Blakemore, A., Waheed, M. W., & Waheed, W. (2019). The experiences of lay health workers trained in task-shifting psychological interventions: A qualitative systematic review. *International Journal of Mental Health Systems, 13*(1). https://doi.org/10.1186/s13033-019-0320-9

Smail, D. (2005). *Power, interest and psychology.* PCCS Books.

Soo, C., Tate, R. L., & Lane-Brown, A. (2011). A systematic review of acceptance and commitment therapy (ACT) for managing anxiety: Applicability for people with acquired brain injury? *Brain Impairment, 12*(1), 54–70. https://doi.org/10.1375/brim.12.1.54

Sorsdahl, K., Stein, D. J., Grimsrud, A., Seedat, S., Flisher, A. J., Williams, D. R., & Myer, L. (2009). Traditional healers in the treatment of common mental disorders in South Africa. *The Journal of Nervous and Mental Disease, 197*(6), 434–441. https://doi.org/10.1097/NMD.0b013e3181a61dbc

Stewart, C., Ebert, B., & Bockarie, H. (2017) *Commit and act* in Sierra Leone. In: R. White, S. Jain, D. Orr, & U. Read (Eds.), *The Palgrave handbook of sociocultural perspectives on global mental health.* Palgrave Macmillan. https://doi.org/10.1057/978-1-137-39510-8_31

Strong, K., Mathers, C., & Bonita, R. (2007). Preventing stroke: Saving lives around the world. *The Lancet Neurology, 6*(2), 182–187. https://doi.org/10.1016/s1474-4422(07)70031-5

Sue, D. W., & Sue, D. (2003). *Counseling the culturally diverse: Theory and practice* (4th ed.). John Wiley.

Uganda Bureau of Statistics. (2016). *The national population and housing census 2014 – Main report.* https://unstats.un.org/unsd/demographic/sources/census/wphc/Uganda/UGA-2016-05-23.pdf

UK Government. (2021). *Detentions under the Mental Health Act.* www.ethnicity-facts-figures.service.gov.uk/health/mental-health/detentions-under-the-mental-health-act/latest#main-facts-and-figures

UNICEF. (2019). The extent and nature of multidimensional child poverty and deprivation. UBOS. www.poverty.ac.uk/sites/default/files/attachments/MultidimensionalChildPoverty-and-deprivation-in-Uganda-Volume1-report.pdf

Uomoto, M. J. & Wong, T. (2015). *Multicultural neurorehabilitation: Clinical principles for rehabilitation professionals.* Springer Publishing. https://doi.org/10.1891/9780826115287

White, R. (2017). *Acceptance and commitment therapy in a Ugandan context: Exploring values guided action* [blog post]. https://rosswhiteblog.wordpress.com/2017/05/13/acceptance-and-commitment-therapy-in-a-ugandan-context-exploring-values-guided-action/

Part III

Using ACT within systems supporting people with brain injury

Chapter 11

Acceptance and commitment therapy for families living with brain injury

Audrey Daisley and Rachel Tams

Abstract

Acquired brain injury (ABI) significantly changes the lives of survivors and those close to them; themes of harrowing and painful loss, psychological distress and hopelessness typically dominate the stories told by those affected. Family members often find themselves living lives that are limited, isolated and far removed from what they had hoped for. Acceptance and commitment therapy (ACT) offers a way of working with the family members of brain injury survivors, through a focus on helping people to respond in different ways to the painful thoughts and feelings that are inevitably present after a brain injury in the family, while supporting them to connect with what is important to them and engage in actions that are congruent with meaningful living.

It is not easy living with brain injury in the family. Acquired brain injury (ABI) often results in profound and long-lasting losses for the survivor and their family, affecting identity, roles, relationships, belief systems, communication patterns, meaning, purpose, life plans and hopes for the future. The research literature highlights recurring, complex and ambiguous themes of family loss and problems with adjustment (e.g. Boss & Couden, 2002; Kratz et al., 2017). Worryingly, these problems are shown to worsen over time if families are not supported. We often see a "ripple" effect following ABI, with all family members, including child relatives, being shown to be vulnerable to a range of emotional adjustment difficulties.

Clinically, similar patterns are observed with family members being referred to psychological support services, at all stages of the recovery journey. Often, this only happens many years after their relative's injury, when family members struggle with intense sadness, hopelessness and feelings of isolation and despair. Many family members hold feelings of shame about their apparent inability to cope, or their "failure" to "move on". These feelings are often intertwined with sadness for a lost past and fears about an unobtainable future.

DOI: 10.4324/9781003024408-14

The current evidence base for the effectiveness of family-focused interventions in ABI is limited. Interventions range from addressing family information needs (Kreutzer et al., 2015) through to problem-solving therapies (Kurowski et al., 2018), and resilience-focused ("bouncing back") interventions to support family adjustment to ABI, based on findings that people with high resilience are more likely to cope positively with a relative's ABI (Simpson & Jones, 2013).

However, there are limitations in the notion of "bouncing back" for those living with conditions that lead to permanent changes in their injured relatives. Getting back to "normality" – i.e. the family's pre-ABI lives, roles and relationships – is often not feasible given the typically permanent, enduring changes that are experienced by ABI survivors. Despite this, "bouncing back" often remains an understandable goal for both the survivor and their relatives. This is especially notable in situations where early education and support about the enduring nature of ABI symptoms are absent or incomplete, leading to unrealistic expectations for recovery that are rarely achieved. In addition, input for families is often focused at the earlier stages of recovery, where the emphasis is typically on physical recovery.

Acute or early input rarely allows for space to discuss the longer-term, more enduring issues that may persist. Families may be unaware of these longer-term issues until the permeance of a relative's injury becomes apparent. Early physical recovery may set up expectations about cognitive, emotional and relational recovery (e.g. that a survivor might achieve close to pre-injury levels of physical functioning yet experience residual cognitive symptoms) which prevent the resumption of key milestones such as returning to employment. It can be difficult (or even impossible) for professionals to give accurate indications for recovery potential in the early stages following ABI, but the expectations that families hold can leave them unprepared for setbacks, or without the necessary tools for coping with long-term difficulties.

There is a growing evidence base for using acceptance and commitment therapy (ACT) with families living with neurological illness and injury (e.g. Lloyd, 2016; Williams et al., 2014). We have found ACT offers a powerful way of supporting families at all stages of the injury journey. In particular, we feel ACT-based interventions can be helpful as the impact of the illness endures, in the months and years after acute support services have withdrawn and families feel isolated and alone in their struggle. By encouraging more mindful and conscious action, driven by the things that matter most to the family, ACT focuses on the processes that can instil hope and meaning into lives again.

Applying ACT with the families of people with ABI

Given the complex, distressing and long-term nature of the challenges presented to families as they are faced with the impact of ABI on all aspects of daily life, it is unsurprising that they can struggle psychologically and become caught up in unhelpful ways of thinking and behaving. Families of ABI survivors face challenges from the outset of the ABI journey; first they have to cope with the sudden and unexpected illness and usually hospitalisation of their relative. Family members typically report fearing that their relative might die, preparing themselves for such a loss, then experiencing relief when the relative survives. They experience the challenge of familiarising themselves with hospital routines and professionals, having many questions unanswered – or never asked due to their intensely distressing and life-changing nature. These unspoken questions are often only given voice many months, or years, later when the relative is offered the opportunity to talk about their experiences – typically relatives, however, are not routinely offered such opportunities. In particular, child relatives of people with brain injuries are usually "invisible" to services at the early stages of recovery and rarely have their information or support needs addressed, leaving the adults with the challenge of supporting children whilst they themselves experience high levels of distress. The same is often true for family members with disabilities or other needs that may see them marginalised – they may be less able to visit their relative in hospital and may be less involved in discussions about their care.

In the early stages of recovery family members face new challenges. These are often characterised by family members as "battling with professionals" – this may involve "fighting" for rehabilitation provision for their family member in the hope that they can be restored to how they were prior to the illness or injury. Rehabilitation, however, brings its own challenges for family members. Expectations of recovery can be challenged as the family are presented with their loved one's new difficulties, and as education about brain injury begins to map on to the changes they are seeing in their relative. For many, hope can begin to fade. Some family members rise to this challenge with a "fight" response – they can become determined to prove professionals wrong, struggle to accept the prognostic predictions being offered and work relentlessly to help their relative "beat" the brain injury. Families face the challenge of understanding and knowing how best to respond to and cope with the changes in their loved one. Research tells us that family members "accept" physical limitations more readily than those that occur as a result of changes to cognition, personality and behaviour. Longer-term challenges for the family include finding a way to live with, accept (if this is ever fully possible) and love the "stranger" that is their altered family member (Kreutzer et al., 2015).

As humans we are continually attempting to problem-solve and minimise pain and suffering in our lives. Given the challenges outlined above, it is therefore understandable that family members often respond to ABI-related challenges by attempting to avoid or control the painful thoughts and feelings aroused. Alternatively, they may invest all of their energy into trying to solve or "cure" their relative's injury, or their emotional responses to the consequences of it. A key concept of ACT is the "workability" of these actions. There are no right or wrong ways of thinking about or responding to the challenges faced; rather, the focus is on the effectiveness of these actions or strategies within the context of the individual's values. Typically, when coping with life after brain injury, we see family members responding in ways that, in the longer term, take them away from their values and increase their suffering. They can become "stuck" in ways of behaving that are unhelpful to them, engaging in behaviours that in the shorter term may help control or reduce the pain they are experiencing at their changed situation (e.g. neglecting their own self-care needs) but in the longer term prevent them moving forward to live as well as possible with the changes.

To illustrate let us consider the situation faced by Jenny,[1] the wife of a brain injury survivor who was referred to a clinical neuropsychology service. Jenny was married to Tim, who experienced a severe stroke 4 years previously, which resulted in marked impairments in cognition, communication and mobility. They had two children – Anna, 17 years old, and Jack, 11 years old. Tim was unable to return to his work as a gardener on a local estate. This meant that the family lost their home which came with Tim's job. The family moved to a smaller rented house, close to the children's schools. Tim still required Jenny's help with all aspects of daily life. This had taken its toll on Jenny, who was referred to clinical neuropsychology for help with coping with caring for Tim.

The referral stated that Jenny was "not coping", that she was "stuck" in the search for a cure for his symptoms. The referral also highlighted that she engaged with services in a hostile and blaming manner, "demanding" more and more rehabilitation for Tim. However, Jenny had also refused additional carers for Tim, stating that it would be "giving in" to the injury and that Tim must try to do as much as he could for himself. This led to frequent arguments between Jenny and Tim; Jenny refused to help him and threatened that he must try harder or she would leave him. Jenny said she felt "crushing guilt" in these moments, but felt unable to stop herself. Jenny had stopped doing activities she used to enjoy with friends and had "lost touch" with the fun and caring aspects of herself. The referral stated that the two children were not coping with the atmosphere at home.

The six core processes of the ACT model of "psychological inflexibility" (i.e. experiential avoidance, fusion, fusion with self-concept, loss of contact with the present moment, unworkable action and remoteness from values; Hayes et al., 2006) provide a useful way of conceptualising what happens when individuals such as Jenny become "stuck" in unhelpful ways of responding to the stresses that exist after brain injury. Relatives can find themselves losing contact with the present moment and fusing with thoughts of the past. They may idealise their past relationship with the injured person, or become overwhelmed by feelings of regret or blame for the injury. They may be unhelpfully focused on worries about their anticipated future (e.g. expecting the worst).

They can also become fused with judgements about how family life, the world and others "should" be. They may become caught up with an inflexible view of themselves, holding tightly to one perceived aspect of themselves or a negative judgement (e.g. "I'm failing at helping her recover from this injury"). Family members typically experience a range of painful emotions, including feelings of loss, anxiety, distress, hopeless, anger at what has happened, ambivalence and guilt. Experiential avoidance – attempts to control or avoid such painful thoughts and feelings – can result in responses that may sometimes have short-term benefits but in the longer term are self-defeating. For example, behaviours such as withdrawing from others, striving for complete recovery or avoiding discussions around the emotional impact of the injury can, in the longer term, lead to additional issues such as becoming isolated, exhausted, and emotionally distanced from others.

ACT aims to help family members such as Jenny break out from unworkable ways of responding to their painful experiences, to make contact with the present moment to mindfully act on their values. This requires a focus on developing psychological flexibility through the application of core ACT skills and processes (such as mindfulness, defusion strategies, making space for difficult emotions, self-compassion exercises and identification of values).

There is no recognised start point for ACT interventions and no systematic way of working through the core processes described above (due to their interconnectedness). Due to the intense and painful emotional experiences borne by survivors' families, however, focusing on self-compassion and validation is often the most useful place to begin before moving on to work around values. The importance of taking therapy slowly and allowing time and space for stories of loss and grief to emerge cannot be emphasised enough. The use of creative approaches to hearing family stories such as compassionate imagery, poetry, art can be essential for this work; many family stories from the past may be useful or relevant to the present.

Work with Jenny initially focused on hearing her story of anger, loss and fight, normalising and validating her responses and the pain of her experience. This was coupled with grounding exercises to help her connect with the present moment at times of strong emotions. Techniques focused on self-compassion (e.g. compassionate hand exercise; Harris, 2019) and visualisation exercises were used to help Jenny learn to sit with her pain. The importance of being open to her pain in a compassionate way was a theme we returned to frequently throughout the sessions.

Jenny had become lost in feelings of regret and blame, particularly around Tim's rehabilitation and recovery. She described thoughts such as "If only I had pushed him more", and "If only I had fought for more time in the inpatient unit". These thoughts were highly distressing for Jenny and became fused with thoughts of the future. She described how she often thought about the "worst-case scenario" – that Tim would not recover further – and how she felt hopeless that life could ever feel "normal" again.

This was compounded by fusion with critical thoughts about herself and how she let Tim down: "What kind of wife allows her husband to be forgotten about by the rehabilitation team?" She experienced critical thoughts relating to her treatment of Tim: "I scare and threaten him ... he hates me for it", and "I should be doing more/fighting harder to get him better". These thoughts were often accompanied by feelings of guilt.

Jenny also reflected on how the children had experienced the changes in their father, in terms of their relationships with him (and each other), in their lifestyle and plans for the future. Jenny described intense feelings of regret that her children's lives had been disrupted by Tim's brain injury. She worried that they would be "emotionally scarred" from these experiences and that she should have "chosen them over Tim".

After a number of sessions, Jenny also shared that she often wished Tim had died in the accident; this was accompanied by intense feelings of shame. Acknowledging this commonly held (but rarely shared) family thought allowed work to focus on noticing and naming shameful voices and thoughts. Defusion techniques were effective in helping her create some distance from these difficult thoughts and feelings. Mindfulness exercises, such as "leaves on a stream" (Harris, 2019), also proved helpful in helping Jenny drop the struggle with these thoughts, instead visualising them floating away from her and having less impact. It was also recognised that self-critical thinking prevented Jenny from being able to stand back and consider a wider, more encompassing view of herself as a committed and caring wife, a passionate and driven person (a "rock" for Tim). Encouraging Jenny to explore this through self-compassion exercises allowed her to extend her perception of herself to encompass attributions more aligned to her values such as strength, endurance, loyalty and commitment.

Further work around values (using a values card sort exercise and compass metaphor: Harris, 2019) helped Jenny identify that she felt far removed from what was most important to her – kindness, compassion, adventure and fun. During therapy, Jenny became more aware of her attempts to control or avoid the pain she was feeling. She recognised that she consistently acted in ways that were incongruous with her values: "I am not like the person I want to be at all". Jenny also recognised that she had lost focus on her own self-care by no longer sharing pastimes with her close friends. This was central to her identity as a "good friend and interesting person" and connected to important values such as being caring, compassionate, adventurous and fun. She felt that the anger she expressed towards Tim did not fit with her value of compassion and was not the type of partner she wished to be. For Jenny, the intensely painful thought that her husband might remain as he is, that the "old Tim" might never reappear, felt, for her, overwhelming and unmanageable. In response to this, she developed a range of responses that prevented this "reality" from being felt and held – these included denying Tim care (and in doing so denying herself some support), distracting herself with practical household tasks and striving for more specialist input for Tim. The choice point tool (Ciarrochi et al., 2014) was drawn out with Jenny to identify what happened when she became caught up in painful thoughts/feelings, the costs/benefits of such responses and whether the behaviours she engaged in were "workable" and "towards" moves (Figure 11.1).

Jenny began to see that her preoccupation with obtaining more rehabilitation was time consuming, exhausting, delaying the inevitable and ineffective (i.e. an "away move"). She recognised this was preventing her from living well

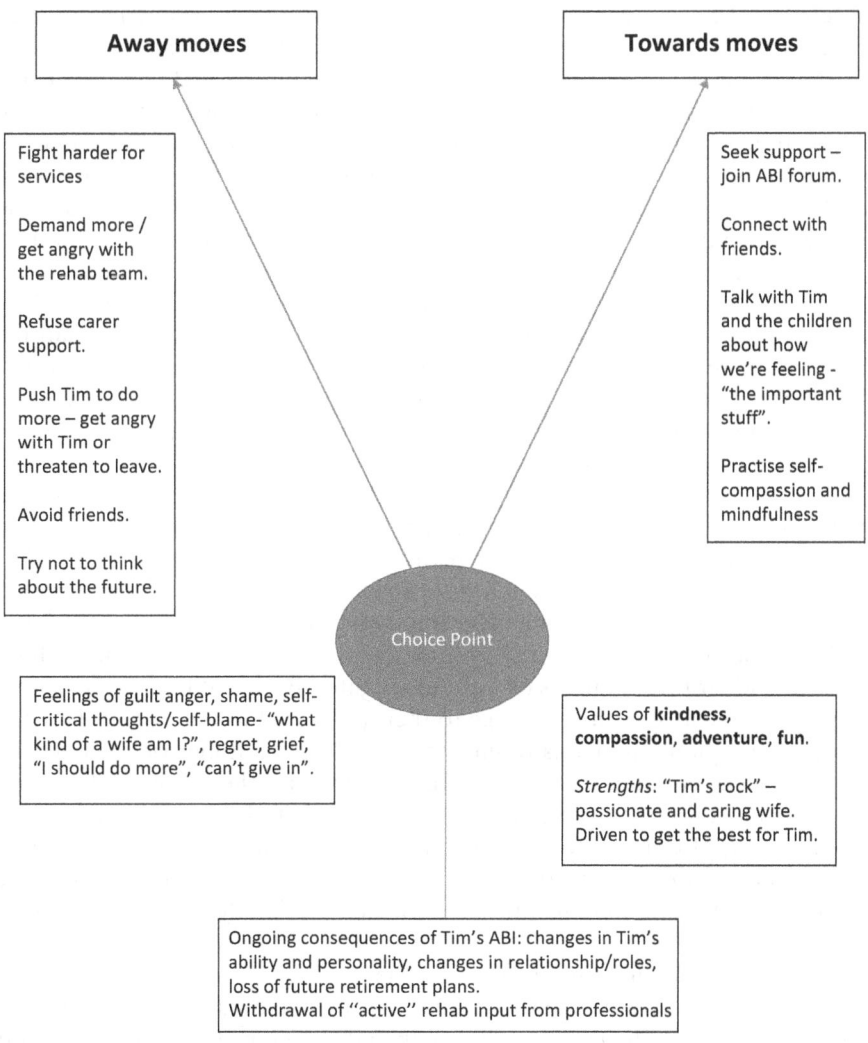

Figure 11.1 Choice point. ABI, acquired brain injury (Based on Harris, 2019).

within what her husband was able to achieve in the here and now. In addition, she recognised that her focus on practical tasks helped her to avoid discussions with Tim about the way they were both feeling, but led to emotional distance from him. She also became aware that her avoidance of friends freed her from painful feelings that meeting with them might evoke (e.g. resentment at their lives moving on; them asking her questions about Tim's recovery). However, this led to her feeling more isolated from her own support network, and more disconnected from her values.

Although Tim chose not to participate in the sessions, Anna and Jack, Tim and Jenny's children, responded positively to the invitation to join later meetings. They were supported to talk openly about their experiences of their father's injury and the changes that had resulted. Anna and Jack shared their distress about the frequent arguments at home and disclosed their confusion about some of the changes they saw in their father. Jack, who was 7 years old at the time of Tim's injury, had held beliefs that he had possibly caused his father's illness; he talked about how he worried that his behaviour at school had caused Tim's stroke, as he had heard from somewhere that stress could cause these kinds of injuries. Jack had come to see their father's withdrawal from aspects of family life as an indication of him blaming them for the onset of his stroke and he was sad and upset about this. Anna spoke about how she felt her childhood had been interrupted; she identified that she had felt a weight of responsibility to take care of Jack and avoid causing her parents any further stress. She spoke about how she put herself under pressure to do well at school and be a "good" daughter, so that she could avoid any need for her parents to worry about her.

Jenny was surprised to hear that her children reported great admiration for how she had looked after their father, and that their fears that he would be "put into a home" were never realised due to her loyalty to him. They described sadness that he was no longer the father he had been, but were able, to Jenny's surprise, to still identify times when they felt close to him. They talked about how he continued to interact with them in loving and helpful ways and identified moments of joy and laughter. Both children spoke of Tim being at home as a positive change to their previous lifestyle, where Tim had worked long hours and was often not around at mealtimes or for weekend activities. The children were supported to share with their mother their wish to be included in family conversations about their father's progress and care needs. It was also useful to consider Tim's voice, even if he could not be present in the sessions. Family therapy techniques such as the "empty chair" and circular questioning were helpful in unpicking the family's thoughts on what Tim might think or say if he heard what was being discussed. This helped the family to hold Tim in mind throughout the sessions.

Over time, Jenny was able to identify "towards" moves – ways of behaving that were in line with her values. These included seeking support from others by reconnecting with her friends and using an online forum to connect with other family members of ABI survivors. She came to recognise the value of sharing her struggle, for example by telling her children more details about Tim's recovery prognosis, and explaining what she had learned about his ongoing difficulties and care needs. She also saw that her continued attempts to seek a "cure" and refuse help from carers were self-defeating behaviours, keeping her trapped in a vicious cycle of "feeling a failure" and seeking more answers. This served to take her and her family away from living as well as possible in the present moment.

Through goal setting within sessions, Jenny was able to set up a meeting with a care agency to arrange regular input from carers for her husband. She recognised that she needed to "sit with" the accompanying uncomfortable feelings that this evoked, for example fears that this represented defeat as it was not "active" rehabilitation, or that it was giving in to the brain injury or that people might view her as not being able to cope. This was supported by discussion of a broader definition of "rehabilitation"; seeing rehabilitation as being about adjustment and coping (rather than solely about "fixing" damage) helped Jenny to recognise that having help from carers would enable Tim to keep moving forwards in his journey towards living well with his difficulties.

Jenny was also able to explore and work on tolerating uncertainty about the future and about Tim's recovery, shifting from a preoccupation on things they could no longer do towards exploring how their family could live a valued and valuable life (e.g. taking up travelling together again). A compass metaphor was useful in exploring the direction Jenny wanted to travel in both as a family and individually – she recognised that moving in the direction of her values led to a shift from searching for a cure to being willing to pursue retirement dreams. Jenny also began to think of care as being a gift to herself, providing her with more time for resuming activities that she had given up in order to care for her husband.

As the work with the clinical neuropsychology service ended, Jenny spoke of the acceptance of grief and loss in their situation. She talked about how she would keep trying to embrace it into their relationship. She described increased feelings of compassion towards her husband, and the family narratives shifted to acknowledge not only Tim's bravery and strength, but the family unit's ability to cope with adversity. Jenny talked about how Tim could have "given up", but instead had endured and she felt now more able to notice these qualities in him; she had been able to remind herself that these were the same qualities that had attracted her to Tim many years ago. The family also said that they now felt able to think about the future without overwhelming fear. Jenny drew on the analogy of the willow tree – that bends in the storm rather than breaking – to describe how the family had weathered the storm of the brain injury. She noted with considerable compassion that they had survived: "we are a bit twisted and torn, but we are not broken".

Conclusion

ABIs change the lives of survivors and those close to them. Family members, including relatives who are often overlooked by services such as younger children or people with disabilities, can experience significant and harrowing losses. They can find themselves caught up in unhelpful ways of thinking and behaving that cause additional distress and misery. ACT offers a non-judgemental, normalising approach to helping family members find meaningful ways to live, to experience, and above all, to have hope.

Note

1   Some real-world clinical examples have been used to illustrate the points raised in this chapter; names and identifying details have been changed and/or amalgamated with other examples to protect confidentiality.

Suggested further reading

Bowen, C., Yeates, G., & Palmer, S. (2010). *A relational approach to rehabilitation: Thinking about relationships after brain injury*. Routledge.

Clark-Wilson, J., & Holloway, M. (2019). *Family experience of brain injury: Surviving, coping, adjusting after brain injury: Survivor stories*. Routledge.

Harris, R. (2009). *ACT with love: Stop struggling, reconcile differences and strengthen your relationship with acceptance and commitment therapy*. New Harbinger.

References

Boss, P., & Couden, B. (2002). Ambiguous loss from chronic physical illness: Clinical interventions with individuals, couples and families. *Journal of Clinical Psychology, 58*(11), 1351–1360. https://doi.org/10.1002/jclp.10083

Ciarrochi, J., Bailey, A., & Harris, R. (2014). *The weight escape: How to stop dieting and start living*. Shambhala Publications.

Harris, R. (2019). *ACT made simple (2nd ed.)*. Harbinger Press.

Hayes, S. C., Luoma, J. B., Bond, F. W., Masuda, A., & Lillis, J. (2006). Acceptance and commitment therapy: Model, processes and outcomes. *Behaviour Research and Therapy, 44*(1), 1–25. https://doi.org/10.1016/j.brat.2005.06.006

Kratz, A. L., Sander, A. M., Brickell, T. A., Lange, R. T., & Carlozzi, N. E. (2017). Traumatic brain injury caregivers: A qualitative analysis of spouse and parent perspectives on quality of life. *Neuropsychological Rehabilitation, 27*(1), 16–37. https://doi.org/10.1080/09602011.2015.1051056

Kreutzer, J. S., Marwitz, J. H., Sima, A. P., & Godwin, E. E. (2015). Efficacy of the brain injury family intervention: Impact on family members. *Journal of Head Trauma Rehabilitation, 30*(4), 249–260. https://doi.org/10.1097/htr.0000000000000144

Kurowski, B. G., Stancin, T., Taylor, G., McNally, K., Kirkwood, M. W., Cassedy, A., King, E., Sklut, M., Narad, M. E., & Wade, S. L. (2018). Comparative effectiveness of family problem-solving therapy for adolescents after traumatic brain injury: Protocol for a randomised, multicentre clinical trial. *Contemporary Clinical Trials Communications, 10*, 111–120. https://doi.org/10.1016/j.conctc.2018.04.001

Lloyd, A. (2016). *The use of ACT to address psychological distress experienced by caregivers: A randomised controlled feasibility trial.* D Clin Psych thesis. University of Glasgow.

Simpson, G., & Jones, K. (2013). How important is resilience among family members supporting relatives with traumatic brain injury or spinal cord injury? *Clinical Rehabilitation, 27*(4), 367–377. https://doi.org/10.1177/0269215512457961

Williams, J., Vaughan, F., Huws, J., & Hastings, R. (2014). Brain injury spousal caregivers' experiences of an acceptance and commitment therapy (ACT) group. *Social Care and Neurodisability, 5*(1), 29–40. https://doi.org/10.1108/scn-02-2013-0005

Chapter 12

Running acceptance and commitment therapy-based groups in brain injury settings

Reg Morris and Rebecca Large

Abstract

This chapter considers how acceptance and commitment therapy (ACT), delivered in a group format, can be a cost-effective way to address the diverse range of co-morbid psychological issues that can emerge following brain injury. ACT may be particularly well suited to supporting adjustment and psychological wellbeing after brain injury due to its emphasis on the development of psychological flexibility and on fostering of value-based living in the face of enduring disabilities. The chapter draws on our experience of using ACT groups to outline how they may be designed and implemented to achieve the best outcomes. The key considerations covered include timing of delivery and content and group structure as well as practical issues and maintaining fidelity to the ACT model. The role of peer support within ACT groups is also considered.

Brain injuries can take many forms, but they have in common the potential to produce changes in mobility, thinking, memory, personality, self-identity, relationships and engagement with everyday activities, including self-care. Modern neuropsychology services have evolved to provide approaches to rehabilitation that are increasingly collaborative, focused on client-determined goals and theoretically pluralistic. Nowadays, there is less emphasis on repeated practice to relearn skills, and greater focus on compensating for enduring deficits using practical strategies and technology (Wilson & Gracey, 2009).

These approaches benefit many people with brain injury, but a significant proportion continue to experience psychological distress and social isolation (The Stroke Association, 2013). Using UK hospital admission statistics, Headway (2018) reported that 530 per 100,000 hospital admissions in 2016–2017 were because of acquired brain injury (ABI; including stroke and head injury). This equated to 954 admissions a day and showed a 10% increase over a 10-year period. Headway noted that no dependable figures exist for the number of people living with the long-term consequences of

DOI: 10.4324/9781003024408-15

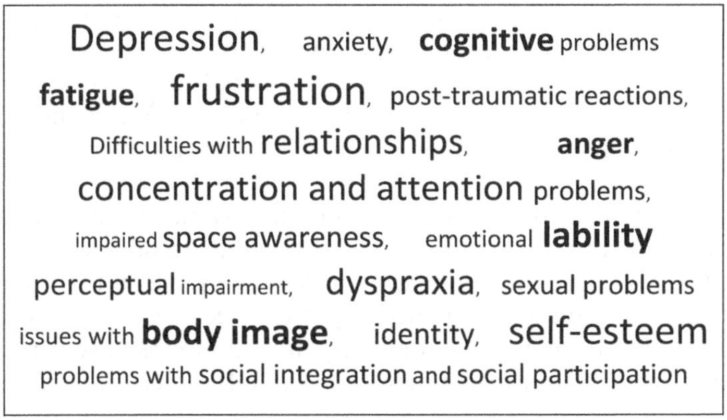

Depression, anxiety, **cognitive** problems
fatigue, **frustration**, post-traumatic reactions,
Difficulties with relationships, **anger**,
concentration and attention problems,
impaired space awareness, emotional **lability**
perceptual impairment, dyspraxia, sexual problems
issues with **body image**, identity, self-esteem
problems with social integration and social participation

Figure 12.1 The multiplicity of psychological reactions.

ABI. However, there have been over four million hospital admissions for ABI since 2005–2006; if only 10% had enduring effects, that would equal 400,000 people experiencing long-term consequences. Including those with injuries from before 2005–2006 suggests an overall prevalence of people struggling with long-term consequences of brain injury approaching one million in the UK.

The scale of the problem is not the only issue faced by clinical psychologists and other professionals working with people who have experienced ABI; the diversity of brain injury means that psychological distress can take many forms (Figure 12.1).

The frequency, variation and complexity of psychological problems after brain injury challenge clinical psychology as a profession. Diagnosis-specific psychological interventions such as cognitive-behavioural therapy (CBT) may struggle to encompass the range of problems associated with ABI. For example, someone experiencing what might be described as "social anxiety" after a brain injury may be dealing with physical disability (e.g. chronic pain or mobility issues), cognitive impairments (e.g. attention problems which make it difficult to follow a group conversation), difficulties with social cognition (leading to neutral responses being misperceived as "threats"), scarring, stigma or a lack of understanding from others (Curvis et al., 2018). Traditional CBT interventions which focus on changing negative evaluations or mental representations may struggle to take into account lifelong difficulties such as these.

Consequently, services are increasingly turning to transdiagnostic approaches such as acceptance and commitment therapy (ACT) that employ a broad-spectrum approach with the potential to encompass a range of different problems. The ACT approach, which does not seek to directly "change" behaviour, thoughts or feelings, but instead modifies the relationship between thought, action and emotion to initiate change, appears to have greater applicability in the brain injury field than the traditional approaches. The potential for ACT in supporting people post-ABI has been recognised (Kangas & McDonald, 2011; Soo et al., 2011) and there is a growing body of evidence to support its use in this population (Graham et al., 2016).

Unfortunately, applied psychology in brain injury settings is a small profession compared to other staff groups; limited numbers of appropriately qualified and experienced psychological professionals mean that only a fraction of those requiring psychological input can access appropriate one-to-one interventions. Many people from marginalised groups in society also face significant barriers in accessing clinical psychology services following an ABI.

Why use group-based interventions following ABI?

One response to the resource issues described above is to use alternative forms of delivery such as group therapy. Group-based approaches can be a cost-effective way to maximise limited resources to ensure that as many people as possible get support from an appropriately qualified psychological professional. However, group-based psychological interventions or rehabilitation programmes are not discussed within national guidelines for ABI services in the UK (National Institute for Health and Care Excellence (NICE), 2013, 2014; Scottish Intercollegiate Guidelines Network (SIGN), 2013), although individually delivered psychological interventions (such as CBT) and cognitive rehabilitation approaches are recommended. It is acknowledged that the evidence base for psychological therapies for emotional problems after ABI is limited and inconsistent, with many studies being of low quality (Hackett et al., 2008). The research exploring use of cognitive rehabilitation strategies after ABI is also varied in terms of quality and outcomes (Cicerone et al., 2019; Gillespie et al., 2015). This is the most likely explanation for why national guidance does not recommend the use of group-based programmes for psychological support or cognitive rehabilitation post-ABI; within this clinically challenging area, conducting robust research studies which meet the threshold for inclusion within national guidance is challenging and costly.

However, group programmes within the ABI field are well established in clinical practice, supported by a growing evidence base of evaluation studies. Forssmann-Falck and Christian (1989) recommended that group-delivered interventions following TBI were a viable method, if they were carefully structured, appropriately led and set out with a clear purpose. Malec (2014) discussed the use of groups within brain injury rehabilitation services, highlighting the potential benefits of feedback and support from peers for improving insight into difficulties, positive reinforcement of effort and progress and therapeutic support. A systematic review by Levy et al. (2019) explored peer support interventions for people with ABI and reported that two studies found significant improvements in quality of life following peer support (out of four trials reporting on stroke and two reporting on traumatic brain injury).

Furthermore, a systematic review of multi-disciplinary rehabilitation for ABI in adults of working age highlighted how the context of rehabilitation influenced outcomes (Turner-Stokes et al., 2015); it was suggested that strong evidence supported the use of a milieu-orientated approach to rehabilitation, based in a therapeutic environment where people with ABI would be surrounded by a peer group of others with similar difficulties. Additionally, peer support groups are a core aspect of the approach utilised by national ABI charities in the UK such as Headway and the Stroke Association.

A further advantage of group-based therapy is that a more complex and diverse repertoire of social skills can be developed, compared to one-to-one therapy (Cicerone et al., 2008). The INCOG guidelines for cognitive rehabilitation following traumatic brain injury suggested that there was emerging evidence that group therapy may be an effective method of delivery, highlighting the potential for improved social skills alongside more direct rehabilitation benefits. In terms of rehabilitation, a scoping review of group-based interventions in traumatic brain injury rehabilitation concluded that most of the studies included indicated significant positive outcomes; however studies around the effectiveness of programmes targeting "real-world" activities and participation-based goals were felt to be lacking (Patterson et al., 2016). Group-based programmes around understanding brain injury, managing cognitive problems and psychological support are discussed in Wilson et al. (2009).

ACT group interventions are an effective way of supporting people with emotional problems. A systematic review of ACT-based group interventions (Coto-Lesmes et al., 2020) showed that ACT was as useful as other approaches. Increase in psychological flexibility was proposed as the main mechanism of change; this is highly relevant to an ABI population. A review of the literature (Marshall, 2018) identified ten distinct therapeutic group processes stemming from peer interactions that enhance wellbeing and help to reduce distress (Box 12.1). These could be incorporated into an ACT-based group for people following ABI.

Box 12.1 Therapeutic group processes

Domain
Instilling hope through exposure to success of other group members
Positive social comparison. Feelings of doing well and achieving things in comparison to what might have been
Unconditional positive regard and acceptance from other group members
Affirmation of actions taken and feelings
Validation of a person's self and personhood
Encouragement to do things and achieve goals
Normalisation of feelings, thoughts and actions
Mutual reciprocity; feeling helped and feeling helpful to others
Reflection/reappraisal of trauma and disability facilitated by peer interaction
A sense of belonging to the group

Adapted from Marshall (2018).

Considerations for running ACT groups in brain injury settings

ACT-based groups have the potential to balance the benefits of peer support-based groups and the therapeutic milieu seen in cognitive rehabilitation settings. Majumdar and Morris (2018) evaluated the efficacy of a group-based ACT for stroke survivors, finding that depression was significantly reduced. Self-rated health status and hopefulness were increased, to a greater degree than a treatment-as-usual control group.

However, given the limited research evidence for efficacy and the complexity of running groups with people with ABI, careful consideration needs to be given to a range of factors.

Timing of the group

The question of "when" to run an ACT group after brain injury is an important one. No set guidance appears to exist around the most appropriate time to deliver a group. However, individual differences around ABI and recovery should be thought about carefully. The heterogeneity and complexity of residual symptoms, degree of disability and individual differences in resilience and coping ability may all contribute to a person's appropriateness and readiness to engage in an ACT therapy group.

Duration since injury may also be a factor that influences engagement and commitment to a psychological intervention. People who are newly diagnosed may place more emphasis on being medically stabilised and their physical recovery compared to those who are further into the rehabilitative process. Although this makes sense in evolutionary terms of promoting survival, focusing heavily on physical aspects can often mean psychological and emotional aspects of living with brain injury remain overlooked. It is possible that individuals with brain injury will not fully process the psychological or emotional impact of their condition until their physical rehabilitation has ended. In our experience, this means that structured ACT groups have been more suited to the post-acute phase of rehabilitation, after people have been discharged from hospital.

Determining suitability for group input

ACT can be particularly suitable for people in close contact with their pain, fused to negative thoughts and engaging in pervasive avoidant behaviours. To determine suitability in the context of the therapeutic challenges that present around brain injury, it may be useful for facilitators to offer a preliminary assessment. Gathering information about residual difficulties, having open discussions about expectations and gauging the readiness/willingness of survivors to sit with unpleasant experiences and practise new skills to manage their distress are important. This can help to determine whether now is the right time for that individual to attend a group, and whether that individual will be able to engage with the group process. It is also necessary to acknowledge the importance of natural adjustment trajectories and the stages individuals may move through as they come to terms with or make sense of their injury and its implications for the future. A fine balance needs to be achieved between not pathologising difficulties that may arise as individuals process their current circumstances and offering a timely intervention to help manage emotional distress that has become problematic for the individual or their family. It may be that individual or family work is required first to support future readiness to engage in a group-based intervention.

In addition, facilitators need to consider the appropriateness of the group format for the individual with a brain injury. Metacognitive strategies (e.g. acceptance-based exercises) require a certain level of cognitive awareness and flexibility, and difficulties with cognition, language and executive functioning may make this more challenging (Kangas & McDonald, 2011). It is important to consider whether the psychological concepts and skills being discussed in the group could be navigated, understood and applied effectively by the individual; this is particularly important in ABI where there can be varying degrees of cognitive or language impairment.

Due to the relative infancy of ACT research within ABI settings, it is difficult to give specific recommendations about suitability and appropriateness for group interventions. Clinical judgement around whether an individual is cognitively able to participate in the intervention is required. Ideally, group members should have the cognitive capacity to retain group materials, as well as consolidate and generalise skills across contexts. One study recommended ACT-based interventions for mild to moderate brain injury, with individuals who have levels of cognitive functioning within 95% (1.65 sd) of the normative average on standardised measures of memory, language and executive functioning (Kangas & McDonald, 2011). Further empirical research is warranted to understand the applications of ACT with ABI survivors with more severe cognitive impairment (see Chapter 8 for further discussion).

Use of appropriate cognitive screening tools (e.g. the Montreal Cognitive Assessment (MoCA; Nasreddine et al., 2005) or the Oxford Cognitive Screen (OCS; Demeyere et al., 2015), broader neuropsychological assessment or observations of the individual prior to offering a group intervention should support this process of determining suitability. Consideration should also be given to other kinds of impairments that may affect the group process (e.g. impulsivity/disinhibition) or the individual's ability to practically engage with it (e.g. severe pain, significant attention problems). Although some adaptations can be made around physical and cognitive impairments (see below), clinicians need to be mindful of how such difficulties may impact upon group dynamics and on the individual themselves if they are unable to follow the group content (e.g. heightened distress).

Designing an ACT-based group for people with ABI

Structure of the group

ACT follows six core therapeutic processes, with each area building sequentially on the next (Hayes et al., 2006). Before introducing ACT concepts to the group, a sense of safety and belonging have been identified as necessary therapeutic prerequisites (Large et al., 2019). Establishing these constructs in the early stages of the group can enhance learning and practice in this context. This can be achieved through the group itself, including interaction with other brain injury survivors of similar backgrounds, suitability of the venue and the authenticity of group facilitators. Collectively, these constructs help to increase the confidence of brain injury survivors in effectively attending to group materials and applying core ACT skills. Individuals appear to be more willing to experiment with strategies promoting greater flexibility and choice as their confidence grows, improving how they respond to distressing or painful internal events (Large et al., 2019).

Box 12.2 shows our suggested outline for an ACT group following ABI; this is proposed as a starting point for ideas and discussion rather than a "perfect" example of how a group should run. Unlike some prescriptive therapeutic approaches, ACT equally encourages flexibility and adaptability within that structure, with sessions being adapted to fit the population, treatment context or clinician preference. This is particularly important given the nature of ABI, and the diverse manifestation of symptoms or residual disability.

Box 12.2 Example outline for acceptance and commitment therapy (ACT) groups

Session	Content	Rationale/considerations
Week 1 Connecting with the group	Focus on getting to know each other. Explore the impact of brain injury; for example, sharing narratives around the injury, exploring ongoing difficulties, and/or discussing recovery post-ABI. Socialise group members to the ACT model. Share the agenda for subsequent sessions	Getting acquainted with other group members can help to establish a sense of safety and belonging, reported as necessary prerequisites to skill acquisition. Enhancing group cohesion can help people feel less alone and encourage members to talk more openly about issues or concerns. Feeling comfortable in the group setting can aid future therapy discussions. Verbal and non-verbal activities can be used to engage group members with different impairments
Week 2 Exploring internal experiences and how we cope with them	Introduce concept of creative hopelessness and address the agenda of emotional control. Discuss difficulties experienced by individuals living with ABI (e.g. psychological, physical and cognitive) and any challenging thoughts, feelings and/or sensations that might arise in response to them. Explore current coping strategies (e.g. join the DOTS (distraction, opting out, thinking strategies, substances/strategies) exercise: Harris, 2008). Reflect on the effectiveness of those strategies in guiding group members towards a rich, meaningful and fulfilling life (i.e. short- versus long-term)	Use ABI-specific examples and invite sharing of personal examples. Link examples back to group material to help members relate to content and concepts. Use metaphors, videos and practical exercises to aid comprehension. This session provides an opportunity to have feelings/ situation validated by peers and to learn vicariously from one another
Week 3 Becoming more aware of the present	Introduce "mindfulness" and teach skills that help build awareness of the "here and now", such as switching off autopilot; observing experiences non-judgementally; and savouring the moment by using the five senses. "Self-as-context" is implicitly covered in each	Strong experiential components enable group members to experiment with different exercises and to reflect on the benefits or challenges of a task. Use a variety of exercises, not just language-based examples, to aid inclusion of members who are aphasic.

Box 12.2 Cont.

Session	Content	Rationale/considerations
	group session; yet it is particularly prominent here with a focus on the "observing self" and developing flexible views of painful internal experiences and the self	A chance to consolidate skills in session may also improve home practice of skills
Week 4 Unhooking from pain	Demonstrate ways to "unhook" from unpleasant or painful thoughts or emotions (defusion skills) and ways of allowing them to be present without fighting against them (willingness, expansion, compassion-focused or acceptance-based skills)	Experiential components aid skill acquisition. Use of concrete metaphors and videos can assist in learning new ACT skills, particularly given the abstract nature of these concepts
Week 5 Exploring what's important to you	Encourage group members to identify what's important to them (e.g. identify values using a card exercise) and to reflect on how closely they are living in accordance with those values. Commit to setting goals that are meaningful and congruent with these values	This session focuses on taking the next steps forward in recovery from ABI by committing to meaningful activity. New skills acquired over the past four sessions can be used to help overcome barriers to goals

ABI, acquired brain injury.

Group sessions are structured or evolve over time. At the beginning of each session, it can be helpful to devote time to reviewing home practice tasks and skills covered in the previous session. Dedicating time for group members to share reflections may also be necessary to ensure each group member has the chance to contribute. This offers space for participants to reflect on positive experiences of using skills and/or barriers faced when practising techniques, which can prompt useful discussions. Facilitators can also gauge how well skills have been understood and retained and adjust the upcoming sessions accordingly; this is particularly helpful for individuals with some degree of cognitive impairment post-ABI. Regularly drawing links between the different group sessions to illustrate the use of skills and how processes overlap can also assist in skill acquisition and strengthening.

Group structure will inevitably vary based on context and the different needs of individuals within the group. For example, differences will exist between inpatient and community groups, or psychoeducation groups and small therapy groups.

Content and style of the group

ACT groups can be delivered in different formats. ACT psychoeducation courses, delivered didactically with a few interactive components, have begun to emerge and have gained some empirical support as effective low-intensity interventions for mental and physical health difficulties, including stroke (Cartwright & Hooper, 2017; Majumdar & Morris, 2018). Despite the utility and cost-effectiveness of these types of groups, some feedback suggests a preference for increased interaction, more opportunities to share lived experiences and a chance to learn vicariously from one another (Large et al., 2019).

Large et al. (2019) discuss a group format which created a safe foundation from which group members felt enabled to engage with learning about ACT and think about how it applied to their own lives. The participants identified several of the processes listed in Box 12.1: a sense of belonging, encouragement by group members to learn and experiment with ACT, and normalisation of thoughts, experiences and feelings. Comparisons (both upward and downward) with others in the group also occurred and were considered a potentially helpful strategy, supporting hope and optimism that fostered positive changes to sense of self in the light of new insights about enduring disabilities.

Opportunities within groups like these can help validate difficult thoughts and feelings encountered by group members, helping to nurture an environment of trust, acceptance and safety. Witnessing other group members being emotional, sharing their deepest fears and frustrations and exposing their inner vulnerability can also model that peers are not alone with their distress and that openly sharing experiences is not "threatening". However, it is vital to reassure group members that they will not be expected to share anything about themselves that they prefer to keep private. Some group members may express a preference for didactic groups without expectations of group interaction; the facilitators may need to strike a balance.

Therefore, when considering the style and content of the group, it can help to make space for flexibility and discussion rather than maintaining an overly educational focus; offering a structured session with regular points for "check in", reflection and discussion can be a useful way to balance this. One aim of the group should be to help normalise the difficulties people may be experiencing in adjusting to life after ABI. We believe this is best achieved by facilitating conversations between group members. Supporting group members to provide updates on behavioural goals set between sessions can be a good way to enable this. This can encourage people to be more open to listening to suggestions and criticisms from those going through similar experiences and may have greater impact than the same suggestions coming from group facilitators (Prigatano & Klonoff, 1988).

The benefit of delivering groups that are perhaps more flexible in nature (e.g. offering space to discuss recovery challenges, share stories of successes) can also allow facilitators to personalise the ACT concepts being discussed towards specific difficulties raised, draw on "live" examples and analogies or work with distress in the room. Facilitators and peers can model skills that promote adaptive coping behaviours.

Hearing how others understand the group material and providing their own metaphors or examples that relate to it can also help clarify issues for the individual, especially if there are varying levels of insight or impairment. This is particularly important given some of the more abstract and meta-cognitive components of ACT; difficulty grasping abstract concepts such as defusion can limit participants' ability to generalise skills outside of the group and will likely deter independent practice. Creating opportunity for greater interaction, discussion of strategies and personalisation of materials with peer examples can aid the acquisition of ACT skills and knowledge (Large et al., 2019).

As an approach, ACT lends itself well to interactive processes. Peer interactions, reflective discussions, group experiential exercises (e.g. mindfulness or defusion activities) and metaphors can be used to help bring about positive experiences and therapeutic change to those who are struggling. Contributing relevant examples to support group materials through using condition-specific or personal examples from the facilitators can also help normalise experiences, by demonstrating that distressing feelings are universal and modelling real-life applications of ACT, e.g. how the mind wanders or functions on autopilot, and how we fuse with certain thoughts (Large et al., 2019).

Organisation of the group

Duration and length of the group will depend on setting and resources. Typically, small groups tend to fall between 1 and 3 hours and can vary from one-off workshops to group programmes structured over a number of weeks (e.g. 5–8 weeks). Group size will vary depending on the setting, the number of facilitators and the needs of the clients. In didactic psychoeducational groups, where there is a reduced focus on interaction, group sizes may be quite large, for example 20–30 people. Virtual formats such as online webinars may allow for even larger numbers of participants. For smaller therapy groups, group sizes of 8–12 people should enable opportunity for reflections, experiential activities and discussions. Smaller groups may be required if group participants have more complex needs or cognitive impairments that may affect their engagement in the group.

Consideration should also be given to whether the group is considered open or closed. Open groups encourage new members to join at any time, whereas closed-group programmes invite all members to join at the start. There are pros and cons to both formats. Closed groups allow session content across the group programme to be planned more easily, facilitating an incremental building of ACT knowledge and skills in an integrated fashion, session by session, fostering learning and appreciation of the more unfamiliar aspects of ACT. Closed-group programmes also enable facilitators to easily balance the immediate needs of group members and satisfy needs for safety, belonging and stability; this may increase people's willingness to discuss or sit with distressing internal events or connect with present-moment experiences. However, open groups are more flexible and require less organisation and administration – this may be simpler for both the professionals and people accessing the groups, creating more of a peer support ethos. The nature of the service and group context will be important when making this decision.

Facilitating the group

There should be a minimum of two facilitators per group, ideally with the lead facilitator having trained in ACT or developed experience in using this approach. Prior experiences of using ACT and practising skills from the model "firsthand" not only ensures facilitators are more "connected" to the material, but that they can also track ACT processes effectively (e.g. creative hopelessness, experiential avoidance, etc.), model skills to the group and ensure the group continues to move in an ACT-consistent direction (Walser & Pistorello, 2004). Someone without this pre-existing knowledge may struggle to attend to all of these components and have difficulty ensuring the group remains true to its approach. Likewise, an experienced clinician can work flexibly, whilst simultaneously teaching core ACT skills, to draw on "live" examples or experiences provided by group members to raise their awareness of whether their actions are congruent or incongruent with ACT and values-based living. Regular use of ACT supervision is also important in maintaining fidelity to the model. Facilitators should also be experienced in managing group dynamics and working with people with cognitive, behavioural or emotional problems that are common after ABI.

An open and honest facilitation style is also vital. Although disclosures from facilitators may not create the same impact as those coming from someone with lived experience of the same issues, it is important that facilitators are able and willing to speak openly about their thoughts, feelings and struggles. Within an ACT framework, this kind of self-disclosure can help to reflect the "common human experience" elements that are crucial to the process. Facilitators also play a vital role in managing intra-group processes and engineering opportunities for group members to share experiential knowledge.

Outcome measurement

A qualitative study of group-based memory rehabilitation for people with neurological disabilities (Chouliara & Lincoln, 2016) highlighted how participants appreciated getting new information on their brain injury and memory function, and improvements in insight, self-efficacy and control were reported. It was reported that although memory function did not improve directly, participants felt better able to manage and cope with their difficulties; this study highlights the importance of carefully considering the outcome measure used within studies exploring the effectiveness and efficacy of group-based cognitive rehabilitation programmes post-ABI. Consideration should be given to what would constitute meaningful evaluation – an overly narrow focus on symptom reduction is unlikely to be useful. Facilitators should also consider whether group members will be able to complete more conceptually abstract outcome measures, such as those assessing constructs like psychological flexibility.

Adapting a group for people with ABI

Knowledge of brain injury, its consequences and aspects that influence recovery is key to understanding how best to provide an intervention that appropriately meets the needs of the population. People with ABI can experience a wide range of cognitive and physical problems, therefore it is important to be sensitive and responsive to the needs of the individual members. Adaptations will most likely be needed to account for the sequelae of ABI symptoms; necessary adaptations should be considered from the outset and seen as a crucial part of running a group, not an afterthought.

In this section of the chapter, we offer suggested starting points for practical adjustments that may be needed. Group structure and content should be co-constructed with service user representatives or stakeholders, and facilitators should make efforts to check in with group members regularly to identify any other adaptations required. Making specific adaptations to account for these practical issues can facilitate group learning and enjoyment and create environments that are inclusive and which minimise distraction and discomfort.

Complexity of material

To support ABI populations in acquiring and applying ACT knowledge, facilitators need to creatively consider ways of simplifying and consolidating group material (especially to aid recall for individuals with cognitive impairment, fatigue or pain problems). This might include the use of group tasks, different teaching modalities (e.g. videos, diagrams, metaphors, etc.), regularly reviewing material from previous weeks and repetition of content or experiential exercises. The inclusion of weekly homework activities across ACT groups can further help to alleviate pressure on cognitive reserves and distress associated with learning and memory deficits. This can assist in reducing cognitive demands and help individuals to manage difficulties with attention and memory. Language should be kept free of jargon and technical terminology.

Venue appropriateness

Facilitators should review the environment in their chosen venue to ensure that it meets the needs of group members. This should include a review of venue accessibility, in terms of access for those using wheelchairs or mobility aids. Appropriate toilet facilities and seating arrangements (particularly to support those in pain) are vital. Ongoing physical disability or cognitive difficulties post-ABI may mean some individuals need to surrender their driving licence, and are now reliant on carers/relatives or public transport. Consider whether there are good transport links or community transport options to your chosen venue. In some cases, small grants may be available from local clinical networks to fund taxis.

Consider environmental factors such as how busy or noisy the room is, as people with cognitive problems may find it difficult to concentrate in distracting settings. The needs of people with sensory sensitivities (e.g. to light, temperature, noise, etc.) or sensory impairments (e.g. hemianopia) should also be considered. It may be necessary to conduct risk assessments and develop plans for emergency input for individual clients (e.g. emergency alarms and ambulance accessibility when working with people who experience seizures).

Adapting materials

Handouts can support homework tasks and practice of ACT skills, placing less demands on memory during the group. Degree of cognitive impairment will vary between individuals; however, generally, facilitators should consider providing easy-to-read handouts that can be understood by the individual with ABI and supporting family members. Consideration should be given to accessibility of any written material in terms of reading level complexity, layout/design and language/adaptations needed (e.g. audio versions, or translations into Braille or different languages). It may be useful to consider recording sessions for people to watch again at home. Adapted/easy-read versions of outcome measures should also be used (e.g. Psychological Flexibility Questionnaire-Accessible (PFQ-Ax; Oliver et al., 2019)).

Careful consideration should also be given to how group materials will be presented. For example, if using PowerPoint slides on a large screen at the front of the room, it is vital to take into account any visual or hearing impairments. Avoid brightly coloured slides or small fonts, slides containing too much information or complicated animations which may be difficult to process, tolerate or follow. Ensure that materials are compliant with guidance around digital accessibility (Accessibility Community, 2020), for example ensuring that text is compatible with a screen reader.

Adapting group content

About a third of stroke survivors and a significant proportion of those with other types of ABI have a degree of dysphasia. It is important to include them in therapies such as ACT, yet they may struggle to engage in exercises or groups that rely heavily on language. It may be useful to consider a variety of exercises – for example, a mindfulness exercise can be guided by visual or tactile prompts rather than solely an audio script. Discuss at the outset any individual adaptations that the group needs to hold in mind, such as someone needing extra time to find the words they want to say. The facilitators may need to help the group to remember adaptations that have been agreed.

Fatigue is also very common following brain injury (Norup et al., 2019; Paciaroni & Acciarresi, 2019). Groups should be adapted to include regular breaks to help with fatigue management. It is important to be transparent with members about the group's structure and timings of scheduled breaks. This can help to manage anxieties, support members in maintaining attention and reduce cognitive burden. The time of day to run groups should also be considered, with mornings often being better than afternoon sessions. Scheduled breaks can be a good opportunity for group interaction and sharing of perspectives, though care should taken to ensure that some members are not excluded from these more informal conversations due to sensory, cognitive or physical impairments.

Outcome measurement

A concrete approach to outcome measurement may also be required. The success of the group may be evaluated by monitoring movement towards values-based behavioural goals, using visual tools to support people to reflect on how closely aligned to their values they feel (e.g. the bull's-eye exercise: Harris, 2008).

Conclusion

Psychological distress is common after brain injury and can take many forms that often occur together. ACT is a transdiagnostic therapy approach that can address multiple psychological problems and has the potential to be delivered in a group format. In this chapter we have drawn on our experience of using ACT groups with people with brain injury to outline some of the therapeutic and practical aspects of designing and implementing ACT groups for this population.

Suggested further reading

Eddins, R. (2020). *Acceptance and commitment therapy in group practice*. HGPS. https://hgps.org/newsletter/acceptance-commitment-therapy-in-group-practice/

Weatherhead, S., Walsh, B., Calvert, P., & Newby, G. (2013). Opportunistic group work: Service-based and community support group examples. In G. Newby, R. Coetzer, A. Daisley, & S. Weatherhead (Eds.), *Practical neuropsychological rehabilitation in acquired brain injury: A guide for working clinicians*. Routledge.

Wilson, B., Gracey, F., Evans, J., & Bateman, A. (2009). *Neuropsychological rehabilitation: Theory, models, therapy and outcome*. Cambridge University Press.

Yalom, I. D. (1995). *The theory and practice of group psychotherapy* (4th ed.). Basic Books.

References

Accessibility Community. (2020). *Making your service accessible: An introduction*. www.gov.uk/service-manual/helping-people-to-use-your-service/making-your-service-accessible-an-introduction

Cartwright, J., & Hooper, N. (2017). Evaluating a transdiagnostic acceptance and commitment therapy psychoeducation intervention. *The Cognitive Behaviour Therapist*, *10*(e9), 1–6. https://doi.org/10.1017/S1754470X17000125

Chouliara, N., & Lincoln, N. B. (2016). Qualitative exploration of the benefits of group-based memory rehabilitation for people with neurological disabilities: Implications for rehabilitation delivery and evaluation. *BMJ Open, 6*(e011225). https://doi.org/10.1136/bmjopen-2016-011225

Cicerone, K., Goldin, Y., Ganci, K., Rosenbaum, A., Wethe, J., Langenbahn, D., Malec, J., Berguist, T., Kingsley, K., Nagele, D., Trexler, L., Fraas, M., Bogdanova, Y., & Harley, J. P. (2019). Evidence-based cognitive rehabilitation: Systematic review of the literature from 2009 through 2014. *Archives of Physical Medicine and Rehabilitation, 100*, 1515–1533. https://doi.org/10.1016/j.apmr.2019.02.011

Cicerone, K., Mott, T., Azulay, J., Sharlow-Galella, M., Ellmo, W., Paradise, S., & Friel, J. (2008). A randomized controlled trial of holistic neuropsychological rehabilitation after traumatic brain injury. *Archives of Physical Medicine and Rehabilitation, 89*(12), 2239–2249. https://doi.org/10.1016/j.apmr.2008.06.017

Coto-Lesmes, R., Fernández-Rodríguez, C., & González-Fernández, S. (2020). Acceptance and commitment therapy in group format for anxiety and depression. A systematic review. *Journal of Affective Disorders, 263*, 107–120. https://doi.org/10.1016/j.jad.2019.11.154

Curvis, W., Simpson, J., & Hampson, N. (2018). Social anxiety following traumatic brain injury: An exploration of associated factors. *Neuropsychological Rehabilitation, 28*(4), 527–547. https://doi.org/10.1080/09602011.2016.1175359

Demeyere, N., Riddoch, M. J., Slavkova, E. D., Bickerton, W. L., & Humphreys, G. W. (2015). The Oxford Cognitive Screen (OCS): Validation of a stroke-specific short cognitive screening tool. *Psychological Assessment, 27*, 883–894. https://doi.org/10.1037/pas0000082

Forssmann-Falck, R., & Christian, F. M. (1989). The use of group therapy as a treatment modality for behavioral change following head injury. *Psychiatric Medicine, 7*, 43–50. https://doi.org/10.1093/hsw/14.4.235

Gillespie, D., Bowen, A., Chung, C., Cockburn, J., Knapp, P., & Pollock, A. (2015). Rehabilitation for post-stroke cognitive impairment: An overview of recommendations arising from systematic reviews of current evidence. *Clinical Rehabilitation*, *29*(2), 120–128. https://doi.org/10.1177/0269215514538982

Graham, C., Gouick, J., Krahé, C., & Gillanders, D. (2016). A systematic review of the use of acceptance and commitment therapy (ACT) in chronic disease and long-term conditions. *Clinical Psychology Review*, *46*, 46–58. https://doi.org/10.1016/j.cpr.2016.04.009

Hackett, M. L., Anderson, C. S., House, A., & Halteh, C. (2008). Interventions for preventing depression after stroke. *Cochrane Database of Systematic Reviews*. https://doi.org/10.1002/14651858.cd003689.pub3

Harris, R. (2008). *Clarifying your values*. https://thehappinesstrap.com/upimages/Long_Bull's_Eye_Worksheet.pdf

Hayes, S. C., Luoma, J. B., Bond, F. W., Masuda, A., & Lillis, J. (2006). Acceptance and commitment therapy: Model, processes and outcomes. *Behaviour Research and Therapy*, *44*, 1–25. https://doi.org/10.1016/j.brat.2005.06.006

Headway. (2018). *Acquired brain injury: The numbers behind the hidden disability*. www.headway.org.uk/media/2883/acquired-brain-injury-the-numbers-behind-the-hidden-disability.pdf

Kangas, M., & McDonald, S. (2011). Is it time to act? The potential of acceptance and commitment therapy for psychological problems following acquired brain injury. *Neuropsychological Rehabilitation*, *21*(2), 250–276. https://doi.org/10.1080/09602011.2010.540920

Large, R., Samuel, V., & Morris, R. (2019). A changed reality: Experience of an acceptance and commitment therapy (ACT) group after stroke. *Neuropsychological Rehabilitation*. https://doi.org/10.1080/09602011.2019.1589531

Levy, B. B., Luong, D., Perrier, L., Bayley, M. T., & Munce, S. E. P. (2019). Peer support interventions for individuals with acquired brain injury, cerebral palsy, and spina bifida: A systematic review. *BMC Health Services Research*, *19*(1), 288. https://doi.org/10.1186/s12913-019-4110-5

Majumdar, S., & Morris, R. (2018). Brief group-based acceptance and commitment therapy for stroke survivors. *British Journal of Clinical Psychology*, *58*(1), 70–90. https://doi.org/10.1111/bjc.12198

Malec, J. F. (2014). Comprehensive brain injury rehabilitation in post-hospital treatment setting. In: M. Sherer & A. Sander (Eds), *Handbook on the neuropsychology of traumatic brain injury* (pp. 283–307). Springer.

Marshall, C. (2018). *The underlying psychological processes of peer support in stroke*. DClinPsy thesis. Cardiff University.

Nasreddine, Z. S., Phillips, N. A., Bédirian, V., Charbonneau, S., Whitehead, V., Collin, I., Cummings, J. L., & Chertkow, H. (2005). The Montreal Cognitive Assessment, MoCA: A brief screening tool for mild cognitive impairment. *Journal of the American Geriatrics Society*, *53*(4), 695–699. http://dx.doi.org/10.1111/j.1532-5415.2005.53221.x

National Institute for Health and Care Excellence. (2013). *Stroke rehabilitation in adults: Clinical guideline CG162*. www.nice.org.uk/guidance/cg162

National Institute for Health and Care Excellence. (2014). *Head injury: Assessment and early management. Clinical guidelines CG176*. www.nice.org.uk/guidance/cg176

Norup, A., Svendsen, S. W., Doser, K., Ryttersgaard, T. O., Frandsen, N., Gade, L., & Forchhammer, H. B. (2019). Prevalence and severity of fatigue in adolescents and young adults with acquired brain injury: A nationwide study. *Neuropsychological Rehabilitation*. https://doi.org/10.1080/09602011.2017.1371045

Oliver, M., Selman, M., Thomson, M., Long, R., Forshaw, N., & Brice, S. (2019). *The development and initial psychometric properties of the Psychological Flexibility Questionnaire for People with Intellectual Disabilities (PFQ-ID)*. Conference paper: ACBS World Conference 17, Dublin, Ireland.

Paciaroni, M., & Acciarresi, M. (2019). Poststroke fatigue. *Stroke, 50(7)*, 1927–1933.

Patterson, F., Fleming, J., & Doig, E. (2016). Group-based delivery of interventions in traumatic brain injury rehabilitation: A scoping review. *Disability and Rehabilitation, 38*(20), 1961–1986. https://doi.org/10.3109/09638288.2015.1111436

Prigatano, G. P., & Klonoff, P. (1988). Psychotherapy and neuropsychological assessment after brain injury. *Journal of Head Trauma Rehabilitation, 3*, 45–56. https://doi.org/10.1097/00001199-198803000-00007

Scottish Intercollegiate Guidelines Network (SIGN). (2013). *Brain injury rehabilitation in adults. A national clinical guideline*. SIGN publication no. 130. www.sign. ac.uk/assets/sign130.pdf

Soo, C., Tate, R., & Lane-Brown, A. (2011). A systematic review of acceptance and commitment therapy (ACT) for managing anxiety: Applicability for people with acquired brain injury? *Brain Impairment, 12*(1), 54–70. https://doi.org/10.1375/ brim.12.1.54

The Stroke Association. (2013). *Feeling overwhelmed: The emotional impact of stroke*. www.stroke.org.uk/sites/default/files/feeling_overwhelmed_final_web_0.pdf

Turner-Stokes, L., Pick, A., Nair, A., Disler, P. B., & Wade, D. T. (2015). Multi-disciplinary rehabilitation for acquired brain injury in adults of working age. *Cochrane Database of Systematic Reviews, 12*. https://doi.org/10.1002/14651858. CD004170.pub3

Walser, R. D., & Pistorello, J. (2004). ACT in group format. In S. C. Hayes, & K. D. Stroshal (Eds.), *A practical guide to acceptance and commitment therapy*. Springer. https://doi.org/10.1007/978-0-387-23369-7_14

Wilson, B. A., & Gracey, F. (2009). Towards a comprehensive model of neuropsychological rehabilitation. In B. Wilson, F. Gracey, J. Evans, & A. Bateman (Eds.), *Neuropsychological rehabilitation: Theory, models, therapy and outcome* (pp. 1–21). Cambridge University Press.

Wilson, B., Gracey, F., Evans, J., & Bateman, A. (2009). *Neuropsychological rehabilitation: Theory, models, therapy and outcome*. Cambridge University Press.

Chapter 13

Integrating acceptance and commitment therapy principles in acute medical settings

Emily Smart, Will Curvis and Abigail Methley

Abstract

The acute stages of medical care and recovery following a brain injury can be incredibly challenging, particularly in terms of the social, emotional, cognitive and physical consequences. Clinical psychologists and neuropsychologists can play useful roles in acute medical settings to improve care for people with brain injury, providing assessment, formulation and recommendations for treatment and support. Acceptance and commitment therapy (ACT) principles, techniques and ideas can also be used with multidisciplinary healthcare teams to support a psychologically informed approach to medical care in acute settings.

In the UK, hospital treatment for people with acquired brain injuries (ABI) is typically provided within specialist centres (British Psychological Society, 2016). The shift to taking people with major trauma injuries or suspected strokes to designated centres for specialist care has been shown to improve patient flow and survival outcomes, via optimised clinical pathways for people suffering severe injuries (Iacobucci, 2019; Moran et al., 2018). There is still considerable variation in the provision of these services, with some people who experience ABI in some parts of the UK being treated via more traditional urgent care pathways. Local variations in the provision of accident and emergency (A&E) and critical care services, as well as the proximity of specialist neuroscience or neurosurgical services, also contribute to the variation in the acute care and treatment that people receive following ABI. For the purposes of this chapter, we will refer to "acute medical settings" to encapsulate the environments that typically offer this early medical assessment and treatment following brain injury, where input from other professionals is usually centred around the assessment and identification of needs (e.g. A&E, critical care, acute and hyperacute neurosurgical/ABI wards) rather than longer-term rehabilitation. However, we hope that these principles can be applied to a range of medically orientated environments.

Whatever the clinical pathway, people who have experienced an ABI are often treated medically in an acute environment. Traumatic brain injury (TBI)

DOI: 10.4324/9781003024408-16

may require surgical intervention or ongoing monitoring to assess the risk of further complications (e.g. raised intracranial pressure, seizures or haemorrhage). In the context of major trauma (e.g. injuries caused by serious road traffic accidents, falls or assaults), TBI may also be accompanied by other life-threatening injuries. Cerebrovascular accidents such as strokes or burst aneurysms may require acute treatments such as thrombolysis, thrombectomy or surgery to repair the affected blood vessel (e.g. coiling or clipping); brain tumours may require surgical resection (sometimes via awake craniotomy). Other causes of ABI (e.g. metabolic, infectious, bacterial, viral or anoxic problems) will also require specialist medical assessment and treatment.

When the person is deemed to be "medically stable" they may be referred for further neurorehabilitation to support any neuropsychological or physical impairments caused by the ABI. Therefore, alongside medical assessment and treatment, the acute phase of hospital-based care also involves input from a range of other professionals including physiotherapists, occupational therapists, speech and language therapists and clinical psychologists. This acute phase can range from a few hours to several months, depending on the nature and severity of the ABI and the care required.

The neuropsychological needs of people in acute medical settings

Due to the nature of the admission, people in acute medical settings have experienced a significant life event with a potentially longstanding and significant impact on their life. The early days following ABI can be confusing, frightening and filled with unpleasant experiences. Medical environments can be distressing in themselves – hospitals can be frightening, boring, lonely, noisy and uncomfortable places. The COVID-19 pandemic may have exacerbated this in many ways; most hospital centres had to restrict visits from relatives and required staff to wear imposing, fear-provoking personal protective equipment. Being upset, frightened or anxious can often be a normal and understandable psychological reaction to the situation the person is in. The incidence of anxiety, depression and post-traumatic stress disorder (PTSD) following intensive care unit (ICU) admission is well documented (Choi et al., 2016; Patel et al., 2016).

In the early stages of recovery, people often experience confusion and disorientation, as they try to piece together what has happened to them in the face of missing key memories and/or altered cognition or communication. People may also experience high levels of pain and require unpleasant medical interventions (e.g. tracheostomies or catheters). Other physical or medical factors such as delirium, medication side effects and sleep pattern changes can compound cognitive problems and difficulties with low mood and anxiety. Neuropsychological problems may further impact physical wellbeing, engagement, recovery and longer-term outcomes (Ownsworth et al., 2008). For example, many people live with the fear of being at heightened risk for another occurrence or exacerbation of the initial brain injury (e.g. a rebleed or tumour progression). This can drive understandable but exhausting patterns of hypervigilance towards symptoms, which can in turn drive stress and anxiety cycles. Emotional distress and problems with coping or understanding health conditions often prolong hospital stay and drive higher healthcare utilisation and A&E attendance (NHS Confederation, 2012).

Following ABI, people may be desperate to get home and want to leave before they have had assessments or treatment that the healthcare team recommend – or the idea of leaving hospital may be incredibly anxiety provoking, given the adaptations that may be required or the new impairments they may be faced with. The person may require assessment of their ability to make decisions (e.g. around remaining in hospital, discharge planning, risk behaviour, decisions around property and money or decisions around treatment). In England and Wales, this assessment may be completed under the guidance provided within The Mental Capacity Act (2005), which advises professionals to consider someone's ability to understand, retain and weigh information relating to a decision, and then to communicate that decision. Within acute services, there are often differences of opinion between healthcare staff, patients and families about what problems the person has and what help might be needed. The time scale and potential for recovery can be highly variable and the level of further care or intervention needed can be difficult to establish (Rizoli et al., 2016). More subtle cognitive problems that are not evident in a highly structured hospital environment can easily be overlooked.

Challenges of working psychologically in acute medical settings

Acute wards are generally staffed by caring, motivated and highly skilled healthcare professionals, trying to deliver the best care possible in challenging environments. However, the busy and high-pressure nature of acute medical settings can make it difficult to work in a psychologically informed way. The complexity of assessing for physical and cognitive impairments that may impact on everyday functioning – and then arranging any further rehabilitation or care needed – also creates a lot of pressure for healthcare teams. Acute medical services are often under immense pressure to manage limited resources and bed availability, meet waiting time targets and maintain "patient flow" through the hospital via constant discharge planning. The focus tends to be primarily on medical status or physical wellbeing, and emotional, psychological or cognitive needs may be overlooked. The medical model – wherein biological mechanisms are used to solely explain damage and disease – is typically based on curing or "fixing" a specific problem. This can generate a culture of experiential avoidance (Robinson et al., 2004).

Communication is often difficult in acute settings; healthcare staff work in busy teams, often with limited opportunity to work together or hand over information. Acute medical wards are typically not set up for private, sensitive and emotional conversations with patients – a curtain round the bed may be the only privacy that can be granted. Medical jargon can also impact on the connection between patients and professionals. Healthcare professionals often inadvertently downplay the severity of a situation or condition by not wanting to undermine or remove hope, which might be well intentioned but can create confusion and impede adjustment – it can be hard to face up to a challenge if we do not fully understand what the challenge is. The certainty that people can rely on to mediate and tolerate their emotional responses ("This is hard … but I only have a week left") is also often lacking in acute medical settings. Healthcare staff are often unable or reluctant to provide concrete answers to questions, meaning people are faced with prolonged uncertainty around diagnosis, prognosis, treatment options or complications.

Healthcare staff can – especially when working in highly pressured systems or without access to good supervision and support – easily become desensitised to the emotional impact of being in hospital, being acutely or terminally ill or isolated. Tasks which become routine for healthcare staff (e.g. providing personal care) may be embarrassing or distressing for the person involved. Pressure in the system leads to healthcare staff feeling the need to rush discharge processes, potentially creating a tension (both within individuals and between different team members) between the need to maintain service feasibility and protect patient safety.

Using acceptance and commitment therapy principles to support care and treatment in acute medical settings

Robinson and Hayes (1997) describe the Acceptance and Commitment-Health Care (ACT-HC) model, an approach to combining medical and psychological approaches to support behavioural change, in the context of elevated physical health risks, medical discomfort or chronic medical conditions. Acceptance and commitment therapy (ACT) interventions have been implemented across a range of medical settings and populations (Dindo, 2015; Dindo et al., 2017; Fashler et al., 2018; Masuda et al., 2011; Robinson et al., 2004; Vowles & Thompson, 2011).

Although much of what has been written about ACT interventions in supporting medical care has focused on primary care or outpatient settings (e.g. Robinson et al., 2004), brief psychological interventions, drawing on principles of third-wave approaches, may also be useful within acute medical settings (Curvis, 2019). There is emerging evidence to support the effectiveness and usefulness of single-session ACT interventions to support anxiety and mood (Kroska, 2018), health-related behaviour change (e.g. reducing tobacco and alcohol use, or improving physical activity, nutrition and sleep; Barreto & Gaynor, 2019) and post-surgical pain for women who experienced breast cancer (Hadlandsmyth et al., 2019).

Within acute medical settings, providing pro-active psychological assessment, support and intervention early in the treatment pathway can promote coping skills and psychological adjustment, potentially ameliorating difficulties further down the line (British Psychological Society, 2016; Dijkstra et al., 2007; Stanton et al., 2002). ABI can have a profound effect on people's abilities (both physically and cognitively), personality and psychological well-being – which may not be apparent in the acute stages and the person may only struggle when they try to return to normal activities, such as work or managing the household. A neuropsychological perspective early on in the treatment pathway can be invaluable in identifying potential impairments or problems that may lead to functional difficulties; this can provide a more effective and cost-efficient way to reduce disability (and the associated anxiety and sense of loss).

As clinical psychologists with experience of working in a range of medical environments, we are also interested in how ACT principles might be relevant in addressing some of the challenges to providing psychologically informed care, within acute physical healthcare settings. An increasing amount of work has considered how ACT principles might be useful in supporting leadership and organisational change (e.g. Hayes et al., 2007; Moran, 2010). In addition to supporting staff through reflective practice, supervision and consultation-based approaches, we also believe in the value of being embedded within multidisciplinary teams. Building positive and effective working relationships with teams allows for the "chipping in" of ideas to support and steer care at systemic levels (Christofides et al., 2012).

Guidance around providing psychological care on stroke wards (NHS Improvement, 2017) highlights the value of a multidisciplinary approach to assessment of mood and cognitive problems, emphasising the importance of healthcare staff being competent in "low-level" psychological care such as active listening, normalising (not minimising) issues and concerns, providing advice and information to support adjustment, problem solving and goal setting, and signposting for informal support and professional help as needed. This allows appropriate support for people with "sub-threshold" and mild/moderate problems with mood and/or cognition, which will be experienced by the majority of people who experience a stroke. This is a good example of a model which also facilitates the identification of more severe or persistent problems which may require referral to more specialist services such as clinical psychology, neuropsychology or psychiatry services.

From an ACT perspective, this kind of early input can provide validation and reassurance around what constitutes "normal" psychological responses to difficult events, normalising and explaining what our minds "do" when faced with extreme stress, anxiety, uncertainty and grief. Acceptance, as conceived in an ACT framework, is an alternative to the instinct to avoid negative (or potentially negative) experiences (Harris, 2019). It is the active choice to be aware of and willing to allow these types of experiences without trying to avoid or change them (Hayes et al., 2006). By helping the multidisciplinary team to understand the emotional and cognitive responses to brain injury – and supporting them to know what they can do to help this process – we can support the development of a ward culture which is sensitive and responsive to the neuropsychological needs of its patients.

For this to be achieved successfully, an embedded clinical psychology/ neuropsychology presence in the team is vital. These roles should be clearly defined and guided by the needs of the environment. In acute settings, there can sometimes be an expectation that psychological professionals will come in, treat the "problem" and then leave again. Providing informal training, consultation and joint sessions can be a useful way to support and skill up staff to feel confident in supporting the psychological needs of people on the ward. Our experience is that, while the context of the setting can create barriers (mostly in terms of time and resources), most healthcare professionals find this approach is consistent with their ethos and values: "we do that anyway – it just doesn't have a name". Recognising that psychological care is valued and important can help healthcare staff to take pride in these aspects of their work, perhaps even helping them to connect with the reasons they pursued a career in healthcare in the first place.

Experiential avoidance in acute medical settings

Although guidelines for psychological care after stroke (NHS Improvement, 2017) describe the support provided by the multidisciplinary team as "low-level" to distinguish it from specialist mental health input or formal psychotherapy, providing effective psychological care in these settings is highly complex and requires considerable nuance. Medical settings can often unintentionally promote and reinforce a milieu of experiential avoidance – strong emotional responses are seen as a problem, a sign of "illness" that needs to be "cured" (this might even be what drives the referral to psychology or psychiatry services). Avoidance might not always be a bad thing – distraction from emotional or physical pain may be the most workable strategy in that moment. However, from an ACT perspective, difficulties arise when experiential avoidance creates or reinforces emotional distress, or when it causes us to become removed from what is most important to us. This can be a helpful perspective to hold when working within healthcare teams. Rather than trying to shut down people's emotional responses, how can we help them to cope with the situation? This might involve thinking about how they can make space for some unwanted experience, while focusing on what they might be able to change or control, based on their values and what is most important to them.

At the acute stage of recovery, "acceptance" may be more about helping the person understand and make sense of what has happened to them. It might be about connecting with the present moment, although this can be challenging in acute settings, where the "here and now" is unpleasant or terrifying. The emphasis might be on helping the person to find workable ways to get through "this bit" of the journey, even if that involves strategies that might be unhelpful in the longer term, e.g. using music as a distraction. A key role for psychologists working in acute settings is to help other members of the multidisciplinary team to take an individualised approach to supporting patients, recognising that there is no "right" way of coping and being aware of our natural tendency to avoid and minimise unpleasant or difficult emotional experiences.

ES worked with Alice,[1] a 45-year-old woman who had experienced a ruptured aneurysm leading to a subarachnoid haemorrhage. She required intubation and insertion of a tracheostomy. She was initially referred to neuropsychology for "low mood" and the ICU staff nurses were concerned that Alice was distressed, crying and at times experiencing what appeared to be panic attacks. This made her tracheostomy care more challenging. A joint assessment was conducted on ICU with ES (a clinical psychologist), Alice's named nurse and a speech and language therapist. Alice communicated through mouthing words, gesture and writing on a white board. Where possible closed questions with yes/no responses were used. Alice appeared confused and seemed to struggle to retain new information. Despite the challenges in communication, it was clear that Alice felt overwhelmed. She had to ask the nurses for help with everything but struggled to communicate effectively with them. She experienced distressing images and memories of her journey to hospital and struggled with the uncomfortable sensations associated with breathing through a tracheostomy. When she required suction on her tracheostomy, she felt like she was suffocating.

Normalising Alice's feelings and experiences, particularly around common reactions to traumatic events (e.g. flashbacks, nightmares, anxiety, etc.) helped to reassure her that she was not "going mad" or "losing her mind". She found it helpful to hear from a clinical psychologist that these experiences were normal, and that a "wait-and-see" approach to monitoring over the coming weeks and months would identify any specialist help needed around post-traumatic stress responses. Alice agreed that daily "check ins" about this with the nursing team would help her to feel calmer.

Simple grounding strategies that the nursing team could support Alice to use were also recommended, intended to help Alice to "drop anchor" when she was feeling overwhelmed. She was supported by her named nurse to access recorded mindfulness exercises on her smartphone, which gave her an external focus for her attention and helped her to notice and name the thoughts and emotions she experienced at those moments. Alice also highlighted that she liked to use mindfulness colouring books. After liaising with the occupational therapist, Alice was provided with large photocopies and adapted pen grips to allow her to colour in pictures, enabling her to cope by re-focusing her attention on a simple yet relaxing task. A voice recording from a family member, explaining in a calm and reassuring tone what was happening, was played whenever suctioning was required – this helped to assure Alice that she was not going to suffocate, even though the sensations were unpleasant. It was important to do this every time; the nature of Alice's memory impairments at that point meant that she could not always retain the assurances given to her by the medical team in the morning handover. Cueing the staff into this, as well as highlighting the communication guidelines provided by the speech and language therapist, helped to improve the dynamic between Alice and the staff team, helping her to feel more understood, listened to and emotionally contained.

This example illustrates the value of a multidisciplinary approach, centred around supporting coping with strong emotional reactions to difficult circumstances. The nursing team initially identified they did feel not skilled enough to help Alice when she was distressed. As a result, they avoided telling her about treatment/care interventions at the last possible moment to avoid causing upset. The team had even stopped asking Alice how she was feeling, as this appeared to upset her. Helping the team to recognise the value of active-listening approaches supported the team to feel more confident in approaching difficult conversations and able to tolerate Alice's responses to them asking "how are you?"

Systemic working is crucial to help teams understand and tolerate challenging emotions, rather than seeing them as something to be avoided. Emphasising the importance of validation and reflection on relational dynamics can be helpful – it is us against the problem, not the team against the patient. ACT principles might be used as part of a team/staff formulation approach to think about "stuckness" in difficult situations, both in terms of the relationship between the healthcare team and the patient, as well as everyone's relationship with the brain injury. This can create space for new options or approaches that haven't been talked about before. This is very different from the "we've done all we can" mindset which can be pervasive within medical services. This may require some reflection on separating what can be changed from what cannot; sometimes we need to acknowledge and sit with the hopelessness, to show that it is not always about "fixing". Sometimes we just have to sit with the person where they are at, holding on to an empathic, non-judgemental and validating stance.

Noticing and naming what people in the multidisciplinary team already do can help with this. WC was approached by a nurse on the ward, who asked about making a referral to neuropsychology:

> Just to let you know, I was on the night shift last night and the gentleman in bed ten was really upset. I didn't know what to do, but I just sat with him and chatted about how he was feeling – it seemed to help.

WC spoke to the patient, who identified how useful this conversation with the nurse had been in helping him to recognise how his thought patterns were taking him away from what was most important to him. The conversation with the nurse had helped him to recognise that he was experiencing normal human reactions to an abnormal situation: "It's no wonder I'm crying all the time because of everything that's happened this week – most people would feel the same". He agreed that he did not need any further support or psychological therapy – that conversation with the nurse had been enough. This was fed back to the member of staff, who was a little surprised that they had "accidentally" done exactly what the person needed at that moment. Of course, it will not always be this simple – but we can support development of compassionate, empathic and psychologically flexible systems, within which healthcare staff feel willing and able to try out different things, to check out different approaches and to work collaboratively with the patients they are caring for.

Thinking about language

Encouraging reflection on language can also be helpful. ACT is built on theoretical and philosophical foundations (such as relational frame theory (RFT); Hayes et al., 2001) that highlight the importance of language – this can be a helpful perspective to support change. For example, the concept of being "ill" may seem an obvious and straightforward label to apply to someone in hospital. But someone experiencing acute delirium (a common presentation often associated with severe confusion, hallucinations and emotional distress; National Institute of Clinical Excellence, 2010) may not feel "ill", despite having a potentially severe medical condition. They may be terrified or confused about what they are seeing, hearing or experiencing – but being told that this is due to "being ill" is unlikely to be reassuring, especially if the hallucinations they are experiencing feel very real, or if they are confused about what has happened to them. Indeed, the more staff tell them they are "ill", the more the person may think they are "fine", and this can lead to distrust and disengagement.

A healthcare professional using an ACT approach might start with a healthy dose of active listening, validation and empathy, before going on to gently exploring the person's worries by asking questions like, "What's your mind telling you right now?" The psychological problems caused by delirium can last months or years, with significant secondary impacts on families and healthcare staff (see Williams et al., 2020 for a useful review), so simple approaches to reducing acute distress such as supporting healthcare staff to know how to engage and work psychologically with someone who is acutely confused can have a significant impact on the trajectory of recovery for thousands of people per year.

More broadly, it can be helpful to hold a curious yet challenging position around other language and phrasing. How does the team talk about distress, and people who become distressed? When we talk in terms of tasks, beds and diagnoses ("I just need to change the catheter on the sub-arach in bed three"), what gets lost or overlooked? What do we mean by "disengagement" from sessions, and how can the words we use change the stories that circulate? ("Refused a physiotherapy session today, due to acute pain being poorly controlled" easily becomes "Refused physio" when discussed at a handover – this might become "Not engaging with physio" when a team is under pressure to discharge). Though we do not want to police the way professionals speak (and certainly would not want to criticise the somewhat dark humour that helps many healthcare staff cope with the demands of working in such settings!), we can encourage reflection on the meanings and emotional labels that are "fused" with the words we use in conversation and in clinical notes.

Reflection on language can also lead to reflection on power. Another common source of tension in these settings – again, often influenced by bed pressures and discharge planning – comes when talking about "insight". Typically defined as the ability to recognise one's own needs and ability to manage functional tasks, differences between the opinions of patients, families and different members of the multidisciplinary team are common after brain injury. A focus on the word "insight" – a term laden with power imbalances and the idea that there is a "right" opinion – can lead to these disparate positions becoming entrenched. How can we work with where the person is at, in terms of understanding or accepting what is happening to them? How do we support their willingness or ability to hear what we're trying to talk to them about? How can we connect our assessments with what's most meaningful to them? Being embedded into teams and drawing on ACT and RFT ideas in a supportive, non-blaming way can help to facilitate reflection on these kinds of challenges, recognising that people are more likely to become task-focused and less empathic when under pressure or threat, and seeking to support the team to cope with these demands rather than being critical of their responses to them. Systemic therapy ideas are relevant here too. Where does power sit? Whose voice is and is not being heard? Where are we situating the "problem" (Heatherington & Johnson, 2019)?

Values and person-centred care

As discussed throughout this book, getting in touch with values in order to live a rich and meaningful life is a central theme within ACT. Values can be defined as the qualities that we choose to work towards in any given moment. We all hold values, consciously or unconsciously, about the kind of person we see ourselves as (or would like to be), the things we do (or want to do) and what we stand for in life (or what we would like to stand for).

Even in the face of changing or difficult circumstances, there are ways of staying true to our values and taking committed action in line with them, even if the end result may not look how we expected it to. Helping people to connect with their values early on in their journey can help set a focus throughout their future rehabilitation journey. There can be practical challenges in engaging in values-based work in acute settings; many people struggle to write or think in more abstract ways after ABI (see Chapter 6). Additionally, in acute settings people often have little control over their current situation. Their relationship with (or ability to engage with) things that are important to them may have changed forever. However, by focusing on the simplest and most pertinent aspects of what is important to someone, values can play an important role in guiding care. Even when someone is struggling, we can start to think about what is missing right now. "What's keeping you going?" "What's most important to you right now?" "How can we find some connection with what's important to you, while you're in hospital?"

This perspective can also influence the way that healthcare teams can work within acute settings. Even for people who are acutely unwell, confused, disorientated or in an altered state of consciousness, finding ways to incorporate values into compassionate care can support trust, understanding and a feeling of safety. Simply writing "What is important to me ..." on a board above the bed can help maintain a focus on a person's values, promote positive conversations and support relationships between patients and healthcare staff.

Understanding a person's values can also be a helpful perspective to integrate into assessments of people's ability to make decisions (within The Mental Capacity Act, 2005).

For example, understanding that a person values privacy and autonomy might help to make explanations of the advantages and disadvantages of different onward care options more meaningful – for example, receiving rehabilitation at home might mean more personal space, but a spell of inpatient rehabilitation would provide greater therapy intensity and could improve independent living skills in the longer term. This can be especially useful in situations where the person struggles to see the functional problems their injury may cause (George & Gilbert, 2018). Values can also help to guide decisions made by a healthcare team in someone's "best interests" (as defined under The Mental Capacity Act, 2005). Within the context of a healthcare system that is under massive pressure, a focus on values can help a team to feel comfortable that the decision made is the right one for the person – not just what is right for the service. Providing support via supervision and reflection can also help a team to identify what they want to guide them when in a situation where they have to make a difficult choice with no perfect answer.

Conclusion

Having clinical psychologists embedded into acute medical teams can improve the care of people with brain injury. Although we have not described purist ACT interventions, this chapter has considered ways in which ACT principles might be relevant in acute medical settings, to support improved care for people who have experienced brain injury. This can be achieved through a combination of direct assessment, formulation and intervention work with people who have experienced brain injuries and their families, alongside facilitating supervision, consultation, reflective practice and informal conversations in corridors with other members of the acute healthcare multidisciplinary team.

Note

1 Some real-world clinical examples have been used to illustrate the points raised in this chapter; names and identifying details have been changed and/or amalgamated with other examples to protect confidentiality.

Suggested further reading

Curvis, W. (2019). Brief interventions in hospital settings. In S. Parry (Ed.), *The handbook of brief therapies: A practical guide* (pp. 157–172). Sage.
Fielding, D., & Latchford, G. (1999). Clinical health psychology in general medical settings. In J. Marzillier, & J. Hall (Eds), *What is clinical psychology?* (pp. 259–293). Oxford University Press.
Yalom, I. D. (2011). *Staring at the sun: Being at peace with your own mortality.* Little, Brown.

References

Barreto, M., & Gaynor, S. T. (2019). A single-session of acceptance and commitment therapy for health-related behavior change: Protocol description and initial case examples. *Behavior Analysis: Research and Practice, 19*(1), 47–59. http://dx.doi.org/10.1037/bar0000093
British Psychological Society. (2016). Mapping of neuropsychology services. www.bps.org.uk/system/files/Member%20Networks/Divisions/DoN/Members/Mapping%20of%20neuropsychology%20Services%20within%20Neuroscience%20Centres.pdf
Choi, J., Tate, J. A., Rogers, M. A., Donahoe, M. P., & Hoffman, L. A. (2016). Depressive symptoms and anxiety in intensive care unit (ICU) survivors after ICU discharge. *Heart & Lung: The Journal of Critical Care, 45*(2), 140–146. https://doi.org/10.1016/j.hrtlng.2015.12.002

Christofides, S., Johnstone, L., & Musa, M. (2012). 'Chipping in': Clinical psychologists' descriptions of their use of formulation in multidisciplinary team working. *Psychology and Psychotherapy*, *85*(4), 424–435. https://doi.org/10.1111/j.2044-8341.2011.02041.x

Curvis, W. (2019). Brief interventions in hospital settings. In S. Parry (Ed.), *The handbook of brief therapies: A practical guide* (pp. 157–172). Sage.

Dijkstra, A., Buunk, A. P., Tóth, G., & Jager, N. (2007). Psychological adjustment to chronic illness: The role of prototype evaluation in acceptance of illness. *Journal of Applied Biobehavioral Research*, *12*(3-4), 119–140. https://doi.org/10.1111/j.1751-9861.2008.00018.x

Dindo, L. (2015). One-day acceptance and commitment training workshops in medical populations. *Current Opinion in Psychology*, *2*, 38–42. https://doi.org/10.1016/j.copsyc.2015.01.018

Dindo, L., Van Liew, J. R., & Arch, J. J. (2017). Acceptance and commitment therapy: A transdiagnostic behavioral intervention for mental health and medical conditions. *Neurotherapeutics*, *14*(3), 546–553. https://doi.org/10.1007/s13311-017-0521-3

Fashler, S. R., Weinrib, A. Z., Azam, M. A., & Katz, J. (2018). The use of acceptance and commitment therapy in oncology settings: A narrative review. *Psychological Reports*, *121*(2), 229–252. https://doi.org/10.1177/0033294117726061

George, M., & Gilbert, S. (2018). Mental Capacity Act (2005) assessments: Why everyone needs to know about the frontal lobe paradox. *The Neuropsychologist*, *5*(1), 59–66.

Hadlandsmyth, K., Dindo, L. N., Wajid, R., Sugg, S. L., Zimmerman, M. B., & Rakel, B. A. (2019). A single-session acceptance and commitment therapy intervention among women undergoing surgery for breast cancer: A randomized pilot trial to reduce persistent postsurgical pain. *Psycho-Oncology*, *28*(11), 2210–2217. https://doi.org/10.1002/pon.5209

Harris, R. (2019). *ACT made simple: An easy-to-read primer on acceptance and commitment therapy* (2nd ed.). New Harbinger.

Hayes, S. C., Barnes-Holmes, D., & Roche, B. (2001). *Relational frame theory: A post-Skinnerian account of human language and cognition*. Springer. https://doi.org/10.1007/b108413

Hayes, S. C., Bond, F. W., Barnes-Holmes, D., & Austin, J. (2007). *Acceptance and mindfulness at work: Applying acceptance and commitment therapy and relational frame theory to organizational behavior management*. Haworth Press.

Hayes, S. C., Luoma, J. B., Bond, F. W., Masuda, A., & Lillis, J. (2006). Acceptance and commitment therapy: Model, processes and outcomes. *Behaviour Research and Therapy*, *44*(1), 1–25. https://doi.org/10.1016/j.brat.2005.06.006

Heatherington, L., & Johnson, B. (2019). Social constructionism in couple and family therapy: Narrative, solution-focused, and related approaches. In B. Fiese (Ed.), *APA handbook of contemporary family psychology: Foundations, methods, and contemporary issues across the lifespan, Vol. 1* (pp. 127–142). American Psychological Association. https://doi.org/10.1037/0000099-008

Iacobucci, G. (2019). NHS to roll out specialist stroke centres across England. *BMJ*, *365*, 14343. https://doi.org/10.1136/bmj.l4343

Kroska, E. B. (2018). How much is enough in brief acceptance and commitment therapy? PhD (Doctor of Philosophy) thesis, University of Iowa. https://doi.org/10.17077/etd.fvn2f0xx

Masuda, A., Cohen, L. L., Wicksell, R. K., Kemani, M. K., & Johnson, A. (2011). A case study: Acceptance and commitment therapy for pediatric sickle cell disease. *Journal of Pediatric Psychology, 36*(4), 398–408. https://doi.org/10.1093/jpepsy/jsq118

Moran, D. J. (2010). ACT for leadership: Using acceptance and commitment training to develop crisis resilient change managers. *International Journal of Behavioral Consultation and Therapy, 6*(4), 341–355. https://doi.org/10.1037/h0100915

Moran, C. G., Lecky, F., Bouamra, O., Lawrence, T., Edwards, A., Woodford, M., Willett, K., & Coats, T. J. (2018). Changing the system – Major trauma patients and their outcomes in the NHS (England) 2008–17. *EClinicalMedicine, 2*, 13–21. https://doi.org/10.1016/j.eclinm.2018.07.001

National Institute of Clinical Excellence. (2010). Delirium: Diagnosis, prevention and management CG103. www.nice.org.uk/guidance/cg103

NHS Confederation. (2012). *Investing in emotional and psychological wellbeing for patients with long-term conditions.* NHS Confederation Mental Health Network. www.nhsconfed.org//media/Confederation/Files/Publications/Documents/Investing-in-emotional-and-psychological-wellbeing-for-patients-with-long-term-condtions-16-April-final-for-website.pdf

NHS Improvement. (2017). Psychological care after stroke: Improving stroke services for people with cognitive and mood disorders. www.nice.org.uk/media/default/sharedlearning/531_strokepsychologicalsupportfinal.pdf

Ownsworth, T., Fleming, J., Shum, D., Kuipers, P., & Strong, J. (2008). Comparison of individual, group and combined intervention formats in a randomized controlled trial for facilitating goal attainment and improving psychosocial function following acquired brain injury. *Journal of Rehabilitation Medicine, 40*(2), 81–88. https://doi.org/10.2340/16501977-0124

Patel, M. B., Jackson, J. C., Morandi, A., Girard, T. D., Hughes, C. G., Thompson, J. L., Kiehl, A. L., Elstad, M. R., Wasserstein, M. L., Goodman, R. B., Beckham, J. C., Chandrasekhar, R., Dittus, R. S., Ely, E. W., & Pandharipande, P. P. (2016). Incidence and risk factors for intensive care unit-related post-traumatic stress disorder in veterans and civilians. *American Journal of Respiratory and Critical Care Medicine, 193*(12), 1373–1381. https://doi.org/10.1164/rccm.201506-1158OC

Rizoli, S., Petersen, A., Bulger, E., Coimbra, R., Kerby, J. D., Minei, J., Morrison, L., Nathens, A., Schreiber, M., & de Oliveira Manoel, A. L. (2016). Early prediction of outcome after severe traumatic brain injury: A simple and practical model. *BMC Emergency Medicine, 16*(1), https://doi.org/10.1186/s12873-016-0098-x

Robinson, P., Gregg, J., Dahl, J., & Lundgren, T. (2004). ACT in medical settings. In S. C. Hayes & K. D. Strosahl (Eds.), *A practical guide to acceptance and commitment therapy* (pp. 295–314). https://doi.org/10.1007/978-0-387-23369-7_12

Robinson, P., & Hayes, S. C. (1997). Acceptance and commitment: A model for integration. In N. A. Cummings, J. L. Cummings, & J. N. Johnson (Eds.), *Behavioral health in primary care: A guide for clinical integration* (pp. 177–203). Psychosocial Press.

Stanton, A. L., Danoff-burg, S., & Huggins, M. E. (2002). The first year after breast cancer diagnosis: Hope and coping strategies as predictors of adjustment. *Psycho-Oncology: Journal of the Psychological, Social and Behavioral Dimensions of Cancer, 11*(2), 93–102. https://doi.org/10.1002/pon.574

The Mental Capacity Act. (2005). Mental Capacity Act. *London: The Stationery Office*.

Vowles, K. E., & Thompson, M. (2011). *Acceptance and commitment therapy for chronic pain*. In L. M. McCracken (Ed.), *Mindfulness and acceptance in behavioral medicine: Current theory and practice* (pp. 31–60). New Harbinger.

Williams, S. T., Dhesi, J. K., & Partridge, J. S. L. (2020). Distress in delirium: Causes, assessment and management. *European Geriatric Medicine, 11*, 63–70. https://doi.org/10.1007/s41999-019-00276-z

Chapter 14

Using acceptance and commitment therapy principles to support systemic change

Stephen Weatherhead, Will Curvis and Ché Rosebert

Abstract

Although acceptance and commitment therapy (ACT) is predominantly a model for one-to-one therapy, this book has considered how some of the principles might apply to other areas of practice, e.g. within groups or supporting staff. We believe that these concepts can also play a useful role in supporting systemic change and service development for neuropsychology or brain injury services. This chapter discusses how ACT principles might be used within homelessness services, to support people with complex physical and mental health needs as a result of brain injury and other vulnerabilities.

To help guide our thinking on how acceptance and commitment therapy (ACT) principles might support the care and wellbeing of people with brain injuries at a services and community level, we have focused on the role of neuropsychology in homelessness services in this chapter. We will discuss some examples of innovative and values-based approaches to service improvement and systemic change in this field. We hope that many of these concepts are transferable to other neuropsychology service settings, as well as provisions for people defined as having multiple and complex needs. Based on the experience of the authors, we will suggest some ways in which ACT principles might be relevant in considering how to run a service in this context, how to integrate with statutory services and how to develop and hold in mind a service culture based around common values.

One of the chapter authors (CR) leads a psychology in hostels service where her work is focused on the strategic development of psychologically informed environments and trauma-informed care. A core component of her work is supporting staff through reflective practice.

Another of the authors (SW) co-designed NeuroTriage, a service specialising in neuropsychology issues in people accessing homeless services. SW and colleagues, including Rob Parker, Rebecca Forrester, Hannah Iveson, Jacq Applebee, Cormac Duffy and Natalie Leigh, set up NeuroTriage to work with people who are homeless and have had a brain injury, providing

DOI: 10.4324/9781003024408-17

direct assessments and psychological therapy for people who are in the hostel system. They also provide training and clinical supervision to staff working in these settings, as well as running conferences and events to raise awareness of associated issues such as mental capacity, managing cognitive difficulties and addiction. The success of this form of support has led to appreciation of its relevance not just to brain injury contexts, but also for supporting people with complex needs such as compound traumas, addictions and criminal behaviour.

Homelessness and brain injury

Research tells us that people who are homeless are often highly vulnerable, with complex physical and mental health needs. People who are homeless die younger than those in the general population; the average age of death in this population is 46 for men and 43 for women (Office of National Statistics, 2019). This briefing on mortality in homelessness also highlights that drug and alcohol abuse account for over a third of these deaths, and dying as a result of a road traffic accident or a fall is three times more likely for homeless people.

The rates of traumatic brain injury (TBI) amongst the homeless population are exceptionally high; more than half of people who are homeless have experienced a TBI (Oddy et al., 2012; Schmitt et al., 2017; Song et al., 2018; Stubbs et al., 2020). Estimated lifetime prevalence of TBI is 2.5–4 times higher for homeless people compared to the general population; for moderate to severe injuries, estimated lifetime prevalence is nearly ten times higher for homeless people (Stubbs et al., 2020). TBI has also increasingly been recognised as a significant risk factor for someone becoming homeless. In a sample of 100 homeless adults (75 male and 25 female), 90% reported that they experienced their first TBI before they became homeless (Oddy et al., 2012). Someone who is homeless is also at much greater risk of experiencing a TBI; a sample of homeless people in Glasgow were found to be over five times more likely to be admitted to hospital following a head injury (McMillan et al., 2014).

It is not just TBI that leads to cognitive deficits in the homeless population; many people have been marginalised from the education system resulting in learning needs; for some people social deprivation or adverse childhood experiences have had a negative impact on brain development, and for many there is the neurological impact of long-term substance misuse and prescribed medications. Whatever the cause, cognitive impairment is common amongst people who are homeless. A review by Depp et al. (2015) estimated that 25% of homeless adults had some degree of measurable cognitive impairment, with the mean full-scale IQ scores in this group reported to be at least one standard deviation below the mean of the general population. Andersen et al. (2014) identified that cognitive function (as measured by the Repeatable

Battery for the Assessment of Neuropsychological Status (RBANS)) in a sample of homeless men was low across all domains measured by the battery, with attention notably more impaired.

TBI in people who are homeless appears to be associated with significantly poorer outcomes and higher vulnerability. Schmitt et al. (2017) reported that the 61.5% of homeless adults in their sample who reported a TBI had poorer mental and physical health and more ongoing neurological problems, compared to those who had not experienced a TBI. In addition to poorer performance on neuropsychological assessments, participants who had experienced a TBI also showed lower cortical grey-matter volumes and lower white-matter fractional anisotropy values upon magnetic resonance imaging (MRI). Furthermore, the standardised mortality ratio for homeless people who had experienced a head injury was found to be twice as high for those who had not experienced a head injury; the mortality ratio for those aged 15–34 was even higher (McMillan et al., 2014). TBI in homeless populations is clearly an area requiring urgent attention.

Clinical psychology and neuropsychology in homelessness services

Despite the vulnerabilities outlined above, and the high prevalence of emotional distress and mental health problems amongst people who are homeless, mental health professionals such as clinical psychologists are often not commissioned to be employed within these services. There can be assumptions that psychological interventions will not be helpful with this client group (Rosebert, 2000). Additionally, the lack of a systemic mapping of the needs of this population has meant that clinicians trained to work with people with mental health problems such as clinical psychologists, occupational therapists and speech and language therapists have traditionally not been embedded into homeless services. This had led to structures and service pathways with the health and social care system that continue to marginalise and exclude people with these complex needs.

However, increased recognition of the psychological trauma, neglect and abuse that many people who are homeless have experienced has led to a rise in developing psychologically informed environments and implementing trauma-informed care within homeless hostels (Camp, 2019; Song et al., 2018; Williamson, 2017). There is also a clear role for neuropsychology input into homelessness services. One of the core roles of services such as NeuroTriage is to provide neuropsychological assessment for people who are homeless and have experienced brain injury, to identify cognitive impairments and neuropsychological needs. Working with a person to help them to make sense of their difficulties, within the context of a wider neuropsychological formulation, can support their understanding – this process of making meaning and crafting a story highlights the important role that assessment and formulation can play.

Applying acceptance and commitment therapy

ACT focuses on helping people to increase their awareness of their own thoughts, feelings and behaviour, and to notice how these function for them in the context of their life, in terms of whether a thought, feeling or behaviour helps them take steps towards improving their quality of life. At an organisational level awareness of thoughts, feelings and behaviours can be translated into – how do we do things around here? What are our boundaries, structures, processes and cultures and how do these improve the quality of life for the people the organisation work for and with? Combining this approach with a better understanding of why a brain injury might make it hard for someone to pay attention, remember new information or resist harmfully acting on their anger can be a helpful perspective to hold, especially when working with someone with a complex history or presentation.

ACT is also rooted within functional contextualism. Without getting too bogged down in philosophy and ontology, ACT emphasises that behaviours are inseparable from their current and historical context (see Hayes et al., 2013, for further discussion of ACT and functional contextualism). No thought or feeling is inherently problematic or pathological – but the context can make them unhelpful or harmful (e.g. in a context of cognitive fusion or experiential avoidance). This is why, in ACT, we seek to change the context; we aim to create a context of defusion and acceptance, so that thoughts and feelings can become less unhelpful or harmful. This also creates flexibility in thinking that can lead to creative solutions and we can find space to take steps towards valued living. Not all the difficulties homeless people experience are related to trauma, but – in line with an ACT stance – a trauma-informed approach recognises that a person's thoughts, feelings and behaviours have been adapted to their experience. ACT is not about repairing or challenging "dysfunctional" or "broken" thoughts – it is about changing our relationship with them, to allow us to focus on what matters. This feels particularly relevant when working with clients or staff teams who are stuck in entrenched trauma-related adverse relational dynamics, and longstanding patterns of thinking, feeling and behaving in ways which are not helpful or workable.

This perspective also allows us to consider behaviours in a broader way than simply focusing on antecedents and consequences; we are interested in the function of a behaviour, rather than the form of it. Functional contextualism also emphasises that behaviours do not happen in a vacuum and we must look to understand the context. That context is likely to involve practical, environmental factors as well as psychological and emotional factors (Bennett & Oliver, 2019). We need to understand this context from a situational, here-and-now position, as much as we need to understand the history behind it. Ultimately, we should be working towards a goal of seeking to understand the reasons for a particular behaviour. For example, if working with a client who uses illicit drugs, or leaves a hostel that seems to provide security, we might stop considering this simply in terms of "behaviours that challenge" – what threats or dangers (internal or external) does these behaviours help to minimise? What discomfort does this seek to alleviate? What unwanted consequences has this person learned to protect themselves from? And from a neuropsychological point of view, what cognitive and emotional processes might be contributing?

We do not want to imply that conscious, deliberate choices are always being made – as human beings we learn to respond to things automatically – but we can shift the narrative away from someone being broken, flawed or lacking in some way, and start thinking about the reasons why those behaviours became so entrenched, and the functional context within which those patterns developed. Working from a position of there being no such thing as an objective truth or right answer, we can support people to reflect on what is helpful and workable for them. At an organisational level we can ask systems of people to reflect on how and why some behaviours, processes, structures and cultures are entrenched, if and when this is helpful and for whom it might be helpful or not helpful.

Understanding the functions of the behaviour within context is key, before we can begin to intervene in any useful way – for example, by working with the person to help them reflect on the functions of their own behaviour, to highlight the costs or consequences of the behaviours and introducing flexibility and creativity, in terms of how they might prefer to cope with the thoughts and feelings that go along with the behaviours. Helping people to reflect on their values can help to guide what committed actions they wish to take in their life, to find more workable or useful ways of coping. This can be guided by empathy, compassion and fairness. A similar process of reflection can be facilitated with staff teams and whole organisations. Collaborating and involving people with lived experience in work with staff can enhance the reflections and learning.

Creative hopelessness is an approach discussed by Harris (2017), which also fits well within this context. This encourages us to work to understand – really understand – what a person has tried already to alleviate their distress or manage their pain, and then to compassionately explore what that has cost them. This validating approach can help open conversations about trying out different approaches to managing the struggles in their life – a starting point for working towards psychological flexibility, whatever that may look like within the person's context.

To help integrate these ideas and support this "making sense" process, various tools can be used – either with the client themselves, or (with the client's consent) to help a staff team to think through what their needs might be. The "Quick guide to ACT case conceptualization" (Harris, 2019) can serve as a useful framework to support colleagues or a team to think through a client's needs from an ACT perspective. This involves asking what valued direction the client wants to move in, what stands in their way, what problematic fusion is occurring and what unworkable actions or experiential avoidance they are caught up in.

Exploring these questions in parallel from staff and organisational perspectives can illuminate why systems and service users may be stuck and point to creative solutions and values-based committed actions for all.

Alongside this, it may be helpful to draw on neuropsychological formulation templates which incorporate neurological problems; for example, the template developed by Wilson and Gracey (2009), which incorporates a range of factors including brain pathology, cognitive, physical and functional consequences, affect/emotional experiences, pre-morbid factors (e.g. coping style) and family/social support. Although designed for working with people with dementia and their behaviours that challenge services, the Newcastle Model (James, 2011) is another useful framework which incorporates consideration of cognitive, mental and physical health needs, alongside contextual factors around people's social situation and life story. This tool was designed for use with staff working in care homes and could easily be transferred to work with staff in hostel services.

Of course, all of the above needs to be built around values – relationships built on collaboration and trust must be at the heart of any psychological work that could develop. Prioritising and valuing the time this takes to develop must be embedded into the fabric of the service. The connections that develop through these relationships between a service user and a professional (or indeed, between different service users) are the foundation for steps towards flexibility and change.

As an example, a clinical psychologist with NeuroTriage (SW) had been working with a client for some time – SW had been trying to support the client to get a mental health advocate, but the client was unsure and did not see what value this would have. SW was able to ask the client if she would allow the advocate to come and meet them in a park – just to come and have a chat. After some silliness and joking around – connecting a little as people – an honest conversation was had about trust. SW said:

> You've told me that you trust me and I believe that you've let me have some of that trust. I trust this other person [the advocate] because we've had a few conversations now that make me think she cares and she wants to do her job. The trust that you've put in me ... can I give some of it to her and see what she does with it?

These connections, these existential, psychological, human links between people, are what leads to positive change. The work is always about people; it's always about relationships.

Establishing values-led services

Considering the broader provision of psychological support within homelessness services, Pathway (2020) offers a clear argument for the integration of psychologists into leadership roles within these settings, to be involved in the configuration of how services are provided. There are various reasons why traditional models of psychology service delivery do not meet the needs of people in this population. Accessing care or health services can be challenging; although people are entitled to register with a general practitioner (GP) without a permanent address or identification, many professionals and service users are not aware of this (Healthwatch, 2018). This can impede access to neuropsychological and other psychological services as well as medication management, health reviews and onward referral to statutory services. Furthermore, standard mental health and neuropsychology services are often not set up to meet the needs of people who may be unable to attend regular appointments or engage in typical psychological assessment or therapy.

When working with people who move between different geographical areas or do not have a regular GP, services must take a more flexible approach. This may involve working outside of normal parameters for inclusion criteria and more innovative funding arrangements from commissioners than the usual locality-based model. In establishing psychological support within homelessness services, it is useful to consider the service level values which can be embedded within the organisation from the outset, and used to guide difficult decisions or highlight challenges to professionals or service pathways that are not familiar with the needs of this population. In the past services hid behind the face validity of the Maslow Hierarchy of Needs model – assuming that homeless people needed to be physically homed before health interventions were given. This assumption is not borne out (Rosebert, 2000). However, an increasing number of health organisations are taking the "no wrong door" approach in line with NHS RightCare commissioning (NHS England, 2018), actively seeking to reduce barriers and increase access to services.

Being explicit about values around equality, equity, access and empathy is helpful in supporting arguments for flexibility and effective person-centred care, influencing organisations committing to valued actions for sustainability and/or change. Most homeless people have had traumatic experiences at some point in their lives. Many staff in the sector have experienced the consequences of this first-hand, making this a complex field to work in. It can be difficult, emotional, time-consuming work that many (already overstretched) services do not have capacity to offer. It can feel like accident and emergency, mental health services, learning disability services, social services and the hostel system are not able to meet the needs of homeless people together – as a result, people are forced through the cracks between service provision and are repeatedly rejected and excluded. By facilitating case conferences and learning forums within and between services and organisations, we can bring the focus back to common values and work to shift organisational priorities. Change can be achieved by identifying what professionals across services have in common and by being explicit in how they might work together.

Pathway (2020) highlights how the problems facing homeless people are not the fault of the individual, or the fault of services which have typically not been designed for the needs of the homeless. It can be more useful to conceptualise problems within the interactions between the individual and services; understood within the past and present social, cultural and political contexts within which these interactions have occurred. This highlights the importance of solutions that integrate interventions around medical and housing needs, alongside embedded psychologically informed care facilitated by employment of staff trained to deliver on psychologically informed environments and trauma-informed care. A multidisciplinary approach here is key, including staff from a variety of professional backgrounds in social care, medicine, nursing, therapy and applied psychology, alongside peer mentors and experts by experience.

Providing support to other professionals

Training on issues around brain injury for professionals working with people who are homeless has been trialled. Pathway (2020) emphasises the importance of training for all professionals involved in these services, including hostel staff, housing officers, health professionals and voluntary sector teams, to support the delivery of a consistent approach across varied disciplines. Synovec and Berry (2020) provided a training programme which covered screening for history of brain injury, treatment planning and information around specific strategies to consider when working with people with a history of brain injury. Raising awareness of the specific needs of this client group, and the approaches that can be helpful, is key. Recognition of a brain injury may increase a person's priority for housing and/or increase the chances of being placed in accommodation that can support their needs, as well as access to additional financial benefits and statutory services.

This could highlight the importance of routine screening for brain injury or neuropsychological issues, as well as more in-depth assessment for those who need it. Hostel dwellers may be poor historians of sustained injuries or experiences that may impact on their neurology, and medical records may not be accurate or available. Such is the normalisation and habituation to violence and injury; some traumatised people do not report that they have been assaulted, been in accidents or lost consciousness unless specifically asked – and even then it is not always recognised. Stubbs et al. (2020) also highlight how, given the increased risk of higher prevalence of brain infarcts, aneurysms and encephalomalacia (the softening or loss of brain tissue after cerebral injury or insult), homeless people may benefit from easier access to neuroimaging and referral into specialist neurorehabilitation services.

Therefore, there is a key role for clinical psychologists and neuropsychologists to play in helping professionals working in homelessness settings to understand the links between brain injury/damage and behaviour, helping them to identify presentations that may be attributable (at least in part) to consequences of TBI or neurological problems. The pervasive interactions between TBI and mood or mental health problems, drug or alcohol problems and physical health difficulties (such as infectious diseases or chronic pain) will likely compound the complexity of a presentation. Improved understanding and recognition of TBI as a significant factor in the trajectory of deterioration are vital in understanding the needs of people accessing these services. Mental capacity is often debated and skilled assessment of TBI is an essential component to an accurate assessment.

Training around psychological theories and approaches can also be helpful. Many people accessing homeless services have difficulties establishing and maintaining trusting relationships (Pathway, 2020). Principles of operant conditioning often make intuitive sense to people – if someone has a bad experience with something, it makes sense that they would not want to repeat it. Stepping back and thinking about someone's behaviour or engagement with services in the context of their experiences can be a helpful starting point. However, bringing in concepts from relational frame theory can help staff understand more nuanced or complex dynamics. For example, from a relational responding perspective, we know that people don't just learn through direct experience – they learn through relating concepts. X is similar to x, which is worse than Y. (See Chapter 13 in Bennett and Oliver, 2019, for a nice breakdown of these concepts.) As human beings, we learn through thoughts and language as much as through direct experience – we can learn to be afraid of things that have never happened to us.

Additionally, as we discussed earlier, if we are to usefully make sense of the function of a thought or behaviour, context is everything. Bennett and Oliver (2019) highlight how experiencing a self-critical thought such as "I am worthless" will be more distressing for a person if it occurs in a context of self-criticism, compared to if such a thought happens within a context of non-judgemental awareness and self-compassion. This underpins much of the emphasis on mindful self-awareness and defusion within ACT. But we can also apply this idea to external environments – if a thought of "I am worthless" occurs within the context of a lifetime of abuse or criticism from others, social isolation, poverty and exclusion from society, it seems obvious that changing the context will make these thoughts easier to cope with. And yet, these contextual factors are rarely targeted or addressed within initiatives to tackle homelessness. Training staff teams to think about the experience of receiving support from their service, in terms of the culture and the context of the interactions between staff and service users, is key in providing a model of care that focuses on relationships and connections between people. This can be helpful in understanding why someone might have a strong response to you, even if you've never done anything directly wrong to them. Encouraging staff teams to think about their interactions with service users through the lens of "how did this person develop this way of thinking?" can help to create an empathic and person-centred culture within a staff team.

Clinical consultation and supervision are also vital roles that psychology provision into homelessness services can provide on a more regular, ongoing basis. This might involve acknowledging and supporting people with the challenging and emotionally draining nature of some aspects of the work. Again, organisational and team level values can give us useful guidance here – especially when progress is slow. The majority of people who work into that environment want to see change – it is a very human need to feel that there's a point to what we do. A key function for consultation or clinical supervision in this context is to help staff to think about what is meant by "change" – even if we are not seeing much progress in the short term, what can we do to make this experience more positive than the last? If a person will only access a service for a short period of time, how can we contribute in some small way that makes it easier for them next time? By focusing on connection and small wins, staff can be supported to step back from the day-to-day demands of their role and reflect on their contributions towards a longer-term picture. Much of the ACT work you do with individuals and families you can do with staff teams too – supporting other professionals to be "psychologically flexible" in the face of significant challenge and adversity can be extremely powerful. ACT has been successfully applied to organisational settings as a leadership coaching model – for example, Moran (2010) describes using ACT principles to develop crisis resilience skills in managers.

It is also vital to acknowledge and understand the demands on overworked and under-resourced staff working into these systems. Working in a psychologically informed way may be experienced as additional pressure or expectation on to already overstretched systems, so the risk of this becoming true needs to be minimised. Supervision and consultation can support staff to use ACT principles to think organisationally, for example to understand the difference between a perhaps more defended stance of "he doesn't need that" to "we can't provide that because we (individually or organisationally) are struggling". By understanding that available resources may not match the needs, the emphasis can shift to how services can work together to meet the needs of people accessing the service. One of the chapter authors (CR) uses a variety of tools and methodologies to support this. The Tree of Life (Ncube, 2007) is an internationally well-developed and researched, culturally sensitive narrative methodology that can be used to help teams explore values and align these with the organisation's core values and primary task (Miller & Rice, 1967). The control, influence or park tool (Box 14.1; adapted from Thompson & Thompson (2008) control, influence, accept model) can be used to help staff teams to think through how they can work in line with their values in a collaborative and coordinated way when they feel stuck in line with a complex list of problems and insufficient internal or external resources to do everything. Staff often find that it can be liberating to "park" worries that are outside their control, if this enables them to focus on things where they feel they can make a difference.

Box 14.1 Troublesome issues: Control, influence or park?

The aim of this approach is to align the group's values with thinking more positively rather than negatively, and to concentrate on what they can do rather than the obstacles that are in their way. The facilitator should listen actively and flipchart the various issues (write them on the left-hand side of a flipchart). Check with the group that the list is complete (if not, extend it).

Once your list of issues is complete, go back through each item, and classify using the CIP principle:

- The problem is something that people in this group can *control*
- It is something that the group is only able to *influence*
- It is something that the group can do nothing about (for now), and is therefore something to *park*

Any exceptions to the "problem"?
Write the classifications next to each issue on the flipchart.
Once the classifications are complete, go back through each issue, and depending on the classification, ask the following questions:

- For *control* issues, ask the group to identify actions that they can take to rectify the problem
- For *influence* issues, ask the group to identify who they need to speak to, and what they need to say, to try and influence the change
- For *park* issues, ask the group what they can do to live with what cannot be changed for now, or make it more palatable (it is normal for groups to have more to *park* than any other type – people talk most about those things about which they are powerless)

Encourage groups to commit to valued actions and to have moments of self-agency, e.g. choose when to compliment themselves and others on the good jobs they are doing; make small acts of kindness, gratitude, self-care.

This links into the ideas described above, around a service culture based on values; sometimes, the best we can hope for is to show the service user that the service can be trusted. That might be in the context of a range of bad experiences or being let down by services or people working in them. Sometimes, users of services form trusting relationships with a small number of people working there; while this is a positive step, it can be difficult for the staff involved to live up to their end of the relationship, especially in the midst of service pressures and pathway problems. Reflective practice can help staff to focus on being worthy of trust, being reliable and being "good enough" (Winnicott, 1953) rather than trying to solve everything, heal trauma or change lifelong habits. For the staff themselves, this can be scary – supervision is key in helping staff to notice when they are feeling anxious or like they are not doing enough, to step back from unhelpful patterns of relating and to be brave enough to focus on what matters most – noticing experiential avoidance and focusing on committed action towards values that improve quality of life for the service user.

Creative hopelessness is also a helpful and relevant construct to consider here. By helping staff teams to conceptualise and formulate "stuckness" with their clients, we can acknowledge that what has been tried already has taken great effort but might not have helped. It can be difficult to know where to go next.

> There are so many people who can achieve things in their lives if we can let them know that it's not going to be perfect, and that it's going to be scary … and that applies to professionals as much as the clients we work with, they're as scared and wanting it to go away as we are. It is not something to avoid and run away from. We get stuck because we give a shit, otherwise we'd just be apathetic, wouldn't we?
>
> (SW)

Engaging with external and statutory services

We have discussed some ideas around working with organisations; many of the points raised could also be useful in thinking about how best to engage with and challenge the ways in which statutory services meet the needs of homeless people. This is often harder to quantify. NeuroTriage has, from its inception, set out to embed its core values and principles into the fabric of Liverpool, through repeated and sustained interactions with people working across different systems and contexts. TBI in the homeless population has been associated with higher emergency department use, increased suicide risk and increased criminal justice system involvement (Stubbs et al., 2020; Topolovec-Vranic et al., 2017); this is unsurprising given the high prevalence of TBI within prison populations and the complex interplay between cognitive impairment, social deprivation and criminal or anti-social behaviour.

Barriers to interdisciplinary care that maintain homeless and rough sleeping need to be addressed via engagement between stakeholders, including those in the healthcare system, the police/criminal justice system, social care and local authorities (Pathway, 2020). This can be facilitated through engagement and advocacy – but there are no short cuts to achieving this.

It is interesting to consider some of the barriers to inclusion in light of relational frame theory and functional contextualism. In human language, a word or sentence can have different meanings or functions depending on context. We would encourage you to pause for a moment, and consider what associations go along with the word "homeless". The word will be in a relational network with other concepts, stories, ideas or beliefs – some of which may be (or are likely to be) stigmatising or associated with negative connotations. When we say "homeless", we don't just mean "to be without a home".

Indeed, the word "homeless" is in itself a relational term – we are defining the person as being without a home, thus implying that the "normal" state of a person is to be "with" a home. How does that relate to internalised concepts we have around what it means to be a "normal" member of this thing we call society? The assumptions that go beyond the state of being "without a home" mean that the word "homeless" becomes more figurative than literal – we use it as a verbal shorthand to communicate a complex array of interacting factors, often without stopping to consider that the verbal shorthand might mean different things to different people. It is important to have a homed mind and body; these don't always co-exist easily or at the same time.

These associations and relational networks will have been developed throughout your life, shaped by your own experiences, comments from or opinions of those close to you and wider influences such as media narratives or political initiatives. By broadening these networks and thinking about the role of other factors such as adverse life events, trauma, brain injury and mental health problems, we believe that we can shape the attributions and automatic assumptions and shift towards a position of empathy. Supporting awareness of this across the system will help redefine homeless not just in terms of needs and vulnerabilities requiring a specialist approach but also recognising the strengths and creativity that exist within individuals and services.

Highlighting the impact of neuropsychological impairments on functional activities of daily living, social skills and emotional regulation can help staff teams and wider systems understand what a person is unable to do, or needs support with. For example, SW worked with a man who had been in and out of the prison system multiple times; on one occasion he was found to be in contempt of court and had 2 weeks added to his sentence for laughing at the judge as the proceedings were ongoing. However, this man had a significant injury to his frontal lobes and experienced problems with executive dysfunction. NeuroTriage was able to help communicate his neuropsychological needs in an understandable way, reporting on standardised test scores that could be compared to the general population, creating a moral argument around what "fair" treatment would involve, with a scientific foundation. Having this built into the service framework from the outset can help to create a culture where this perspective flows outwards, allowing opportunities for connection and collaboration within every contact with external services. In highlighting the needs of this population to external services, we can consider three key elements;

1. The *social* element involves sharing a service model that can work, as well as a societal model that can work, highlighting that, although complex, meeting the needs of this population is not impossible.
2. The *financial* element is about making a simple argument; if people are supported properly, the contact with high-cost statutory services can be dramatically reduced.
3. The *moral* element focuses on telling stories about human beings, for example, sharing interviews, speaking at conferences or producing films to help the general public see that this is a population made of people that in theory could be any of us, but tend to be those already discriminated against.

By targeting these three areas, we can act within key values – understanding, fairness, compassion and inclusion, as well as cooperation and collaboration. This can help break down the typical, individually focused ways of working for services. For example, although many people in the homelessness system have experienced significant trauma, they would not be able to access mental health services due to drug/alcohol problems – yet their mental health problems may impede their ability to engage with drug/alcohol rehabilitation. The majority who work in those settings do so because they care – nobody is in it for the money. But the constraints put on staff by the systems in which they work can impede the core purpose. By working jointly and modelling more flexible ways of working, pathways between services can be developed and improved to meet the needs of the people most in need.

Of course, it is not this simple. Sharing values is not enough. Services, systems and the structures, processes and cultures they hold do actually need to change – historically, services have not been designed or set up to meet the needs of this population. However, for change to happen, the system has to allow values to be enacted. Innovation and flexibility have to be made possible.

Conclusion

This chapter has suggested some ways in which ACT principles might be integrated with a broader approach to supporting the neuropsychological needs of vulnerable people in the homelessness system. Supporting understanding through meaningful assessment and formulation, sharing stories and good practice and supporting overworked and under-resourced professionals and services can lead to real, meaningful change. Although there are no quick fixes or immediately visible happy endings, accepting this reality and understanding the context can help us to make committed action towards values-based activities, which can lead to lasting change and improved care for some of the most vulnerable people in our society. Although we have focused on homelessness services in this chapter, we hope that the principles outlined here will have relevance to a broader range of neuropsychologically informed services designed to support the needs of people who have experienced brain injury.

Suggested further reading

Hough, J. (2017). Changing systems for people with multiple and complex needs: Evaluation of fulfilling lives Newcastle and Gateshead. www.fulfillinglives-ng.org.uk/wp-content/uploads/2017/10/NGFL-systems-change-report-Sept-2017-v2.pdf. See also the Fulfilling Lives website www.fulfillinglives-ng.org.uk/ for a range of excellent reports and resources around system change and workforce development.

Iverson, H., Butler, N., & Weatherhead, S. (2019). Homelessness as a barrier to human rights and healthcare provision. *Journal of Community and Public Health Nursing*, 5(3), 233.

NeuroTriage final report March 2019. www.neurotriage.com/sites/default/files/2019-annual-report.pdf. See also, the NeuroTriage website at www.neurotriage.com/, which contains a variety of videos, training materials and resources around the topics discussed in this chapter.

Pathway. (2020). Service model review of UK mental health and rough sleeping services. www.pathway.org.uk/publication/service-model-review-of-uk-mental-health-and-rough-sleeping-services/

References

Andersen, J., Kot, N., Ennis, N., Colantonio, A., Ouchterlony, D., Cusimano, M. D., & Topolovec-Vranic, J. (2014). Traumatic brain injury and cognitive impairment in men who are homeless. *Disability and Rehabilitation*, *36*(26), 2210–2215. https://doi.org/10.3109/09638288.2014.895870

Bennett, R., & Oliver, J. (2019). *Acceptance and commitment therapy; 100 key points and techniques*. Routledge.

Camp, J. (2019, July 10). *Psychologically informed care in homeless hostels*. The Queen's Nursing Institute. www.qni.org.uk/2019/07/10/psychology-homeless-hostels/

Depp, C. A., Vella, L., Orff, H. J., & Twamley, E. W. (2015). A quantitative review of cognitive functioning in homeless adults. *The Journal of Nervous and Mental Disease*, *203*(2), 126–131. https://doi.org/10.1097/NMD.0000000000000248

Harris, R. (2017). *Nuts and bolts of creative hopelessness*. www.actmindfully.com.au/upimages/Nuts_and_Bolts_of_Creative_Hopelessness_-_May_2017_version.pdf

Harris, R. (2019). Quick guide to ACT case conceptualization. https://thehappiness trap.com/upimages/A_QUICK_GUIDE_TO_ACT_CASE_CONCEPT UALIZATION.pdf

Hayes, S. C., Levin, M. E., Plumb-Vilardaga, J., Villatte, J. L., & Pistorello, J. (2013). Acceptance and commitment therapy and contextual behavioral science: Examining the progress of a distinctive model of behavioral and cognitive therapy. *Behavior Therapy*, *44*(2), 180–198. https://doi.org/10.1016/j.beth.2009.08.002

Healthwatch. (2018). *Improving access to GP services for people who are homeless.* www.healthwatch.co.uk/news/2018-03-23/improving-access-gp-services-people-who-are-homeless

James, I. A. (2011). Understanding behaviour in dementia that challenges. Jessica Kingsley.

McMillan, T. M., Laurie, M., Oddy, M., Menzies, M., Stewart, E., & Wainman-Lefley, J. (2014). Head injury and mortality in the homeless. *Journal of Neurotrauma*, *32*(2), 116–119. https://doi.org/10.1089/neu.2014.3387

Miller, E. J., & Rice, A. K. (1967). *Systems of organization, the control of task and sentient boundaries.* Tavistock.

Moran, D. J. (2010). ACT for leadership: Using acceptance and commitment training to develop crisis-resilient change managers. *International Journal of Behavioral Consultation and Therapy*, *6*(4), 341–355. https://doi.org/10.1037/h0100915

Ncube, N. (2007). The Tree of Life Project. Keynote presentation at the 8th International Conference for Narrative Therapy and Community Work in Kristiansand, Norway.

NHS England. (2018). *What is NHS RightCare? Preparing for 2019/20 operational planning and contracting.* NHS England. www.england.nhs.uk/rightcare/what-is-nhs-rightcare/

Oddy, M., Moir, J. F., Fortescue, D., & Chadwick, S. (2012). The prevalence of traumatic brain injury in the homeless community in a UK city. *Brain Injury*, *26*(9), 1058–1064. https://doi.org/10.3109/02699052.2012.667595

Office of National Statistics. (2019). Deaths of homeless people in England and Wales. www.ons.gov.uk/peoplepopulationandcommunity/birthsdeathsandmarriages/deaths/bulletins/deathsofhomelesspeopleinenglandandwales/2019registrations

Pathway. (2020). Service model review of UK mental health and rough sleeping services. www.pathway.org.uk/publication/service-model-review-of-uk-mental-health-and-rough-sleeping-services/

Rosebert, C. (2000). *The role of clinical psychology for homeless people* [Ph.D., Open University]. https://doi.org/10.21954/ou.ro.0000e2de

Schmitt, T., Thornton, A. E., Rawtaer, I., Barr, A. M., Gicas, K. M., Lang, D. J., Vertinsky, A. T., Rauscher, A., Procyshyn, R. M., Buchanan, T., Cheng, A., MacKay, S., Leonova, O., Langheimer, V., Field, T. S., Heran, M. K., Vila-Rodriguez, F., O'Connor, T. A., MacEwan, G. W., & Panenka, W. J. (2017). Traumatic brain injury in a community-based cohort of homeless and vulnerably housed individuals. *Journal of Neurotrauma*, *34*(23), 3301–3310. https://doi.org/10.1089/neu.2017.5076

Song, M. J., Nikoo, M., Choi, F., Schütz, C. G., Jang, K., & Krausz, R. M. (2018). Childhood trauma and lifetime traumatic brain injury among individuals who are homeless. *The Journal of Head Trauma Rehabilitation*, *33*(3), 185–190. https://doi.org/10.1097/HTR.0000000000000310

Stubbs, J. L., Thornton, A. E., Sevick, J. M., Silverberg, N. D., Barr, A. M., Honer, W. G., & Panenka, W. J. (2020). Traumatic brain injury in homeless and marginally housed individuals: A systematic review and meta-analysis. *The Lancet Public Health*, 5(1), e19–e32. https://doi.org/10.1016/S2468-2667(19)30188-4

Synovec, C. E., & Berry, S. (2020). Addressing brain injury in health care for the homeless settings: A pilot model for provider training. *Work*, *65*(2), 285–296. https://doi.org/10.3233/WOR-203080

Thompson, S., & Thompson, N. (2008*). The critically reflective practitioner*. Palgrave Macmillan.

Topolovec-Vranic, J., Schuler, A., Gozdzik, A., Somers, J., Bourque, P.-É., Frankish, C. J., Jbilou, J., Pakzad, S., Palma Lazgare, L. I., & Hwang, S. W. (2017). The high burden of traumatic brain injury and comorbidities amongst homeless adults with mental illness. *Journal of Psychiatric Research*, *87*, 53–60. https://doi.org/10.1016/j.jpsychires.2016.12.004

Williamson, E. (2017, January 4). *Psychology in hostels project (Lambeth)*. Mental Health Service Directory. http://positivepracticemhdirectory.org/archive/psychology-hostels-project-lambeth/

Wilson, B., & Gracey, F. (2009). In B. Wilson, F. Gracey, J. Evans, & A. Bateman (Eds.), *Neuropsychological rehabilitation: Theory, models, therapy and outcome* (pp. 1–21). Cambridge University Press.

Winnicott, D. W. (1953). Transitional objects and transitional phenomena: A study of the first not-me possession. *International Journal of Psychoanalysis, 34*(2), 89–97. https://doi.org/10.4324/9780429475931-14

Chapter 15

Surviving and thriving

Acceptance and commitment therapy for staff self-care in acquired brain injury services

Jo Black

Abstract

This chapter considers some of the challenges faced by clinicians working with people who have experienced acquired brain injury, which by their nature can affect staff wellbeing. Clinicians spend their working lives in the presence of loss, trying to facilitate adjustment and growth where real physical limits exist. Stretched services, particularly given the pressures of COVID-19, present barriers to delivering the person-centred, empathic and responsive care which many clinicians and clients value. Acceptance and commitment therapy (ACT) lends itself well to work around staff self-care, given its relevance as a model of universal human experience (rather than diagnosis or pathology). ACT can provide a framework for understanding natural and common struggles when working in this field, and for developing psychological flexibility, self-compassion and resourcefulness in managing inevitable stress and self-doubt. The rationale for this, supported by emerging evidence, will be considered, alongside some brief practical ideas relevant to ABI work.

All jobs require the development of skillsets, which are explicitly "trained" as well as developing over time and experience. For professionals[1] working with people and families who are struggling to cope with or adjust to an acquired brain injury (ABI), some of these skills sit at the boundary between the professional and the personal – how can I look after myself, juggle competing demands in and out of work and live a good life, while still being able to witness, hear about and be faced with distress, loss and pain? How can I maintain my ability to instil hope or facilitate growth in the face of grief, sadness, anger and uncertainty? Having responsibility for the care of people with ABI (either directly in therapy or rehabilitation or through supporting the work of other professionals) is likely to be especially emotive, given the nature of the work.

The emphasis on "self-care" for clinicians is enshrined in professional policy, training and increasingly in healthcare culture, yet often with little clarity about how this can be achieved. Surface level discussion of self-care

DOI: 10.4324/9781003024408-18

can alienate clinicians, who can feel either blamed (it must be their fault that they are stressed or emotional, they should be more "resilient") or powerless (feeling unable to effect change in the face of many pressures). It is hard to find time for self-care within a context of working in clinical services which are operating at (or over) capacity. Acceptance and commitment therapy (ACT) is an approach which offers a lot to this discussion, given its focus on "psychological flexibility" – staff delivering work they value, in a way they value, because they are aware of and able to respond to natural stress and challenge without becoming avoidant or consumed by it.

To struggle is normal: using ACT to understand ABI clinicians' challenges

Themes arising in ABI work are often very emotive and challenging. Working with illness, disability, grief and loss forces consideration of one's own mortality and the frailty and uncertainty of life and health. Clinicians encounter neurological conditions that are rare in the general population, but common in referrals to regional services; this can give a skewed perception of risk and raise anxiety about the health of ourselves and our loved ones. People being supported by services are often active individuals who were living regular lives, before finding themselves on the receiving end of instantaneous and undeserved health "apocalypses" – for clinicians, this can lead to inevitable questions about one's own safety. Values and assumptions that we have never consciously thought about can be shaken by the questions raised by this work – could I still live a valued life with severe disability or a progressive terminal condition? Could I personally love my partner to the point of delivering devoted 24-hour care? As clinicians working with people with neurological conditions and ABI, the ability to recognise, reflect upon and tolerate the significant personal impact of the role is essential, not only for self-care, but for the self-awareness needed to work psychologically for the benefit of others.

Seen from an ACT perspective, the internal experiences (feelings, thoughts, beliefs, doubts) inherent in ABI work are likely to challenge clinicians' ability to be psychologically flexible. Difficult feelings of anxiety, sadness or self-doubt could lead understandably to experiential avoidance – the "pulling away" from unpleasant situations, thoughts, feelings or sensations. Clients and their families can struggle to allow the feeling and expression of normal grief, without minimisation, blame, fixing or "cheering up". The "work" often needed from clinicians in these settings is to tolerate pain without turning away – though staff themselves are not immune to cultural programming around expression and control of emotion. Staff often come into such caring roles holding values around the importance of making a positive difference to others, contributing to the people they work with or feeling effective. When facing long-term conditions and chronic disability, it can be difficult for staff to feel they are working in a way which is consistent with these values.

Demands on therapists' emotional regulation, and the prioritisation of the client's needs, require a high level of "emotional labour", a concept referring to the management of emotional expression to fit with job requirements (Biron & van Veldhoven, 2012).

Giving oneself permission for "self-care" can be difficult. Clinicians can feel selfish and petty in considering their own needs when working with others in such tragic situations. This can lead to unclear boundaries, experiential avoidance and lack of self-compassion. For any health professional, there can be a tension between remaining emotionally connected to the work (e.g. feeling genuine empathy and care for clients), and needing to have some professional detachment, in order to remain reflective, functional and emotionally resilient with multiple clients and demands. All staff are likely to experience the vulnerability of hearing a story which is particularly "close to home"; or conversely, feeling too detached and closed off when overwhelmed and stressed. There is a need to find a balance in which staff can be emotionally available and able to engage with the challenges of the work without becoming overwhelmed or avoidant.

In addition, the chronic and complex impacts of ABIs may lead to clinicians struggling to manage expectations for themselves or their work. Some clinical issues faced by people who have experienced an ABI are likely to be long-term – while there may be scope for improvement, rehabilitation or compensation, many people experience life-changing physical and neuropsychological impairments. Emotional adjustment can be arduous and slow. For clinicians, this can be difficult to "sit with" – we often want to help, to fix and to cure. Ingenuity, creativity and patience are vital, but difficult to access if staff are in a place of being overwhelmed, rushed and stressed by the emotional demands of the role. This energy is difficult to maintain in situations where progress is slow and success is hard to see.

Staff who are struggling emotionally can start to believe the more negative aspects of their own internal world. They might become "fused" with self-critical thoughts of their own ineffectiveness, the superiority of other therapists or other "stories" they internally replay, causing distress, self-doubt or avoidance in response to ongoing challenges (Colodro & Oliver, 2018; Harris, 2017a). In addition, pressures and limitations of stretched services can become internalised, with many conscientious clinicians feeling self-critical because they cannot deliver responsive, person-centred care, through no fault of their own. Understandable desires to project an image of professionalism and "coping" can permeate unhelpful cultures in teams. Individuals can feel worried or ashamed of showing any struggle, or conclude that their struggle is due to weakness, lack of knowledge or competence – perhaps universal internal "hooks" as clinicians.

These challenges may limit a clinician's ability to live a valued life at home and at work – perhaps through distress, experiential avoidance, stuckness in difficult patterns of behaviour or feeling "out of line" with one's own professional and personal values (akin to ideas about "burnout"). ACT approaches often focus on "living well with" struggle. An ACT mindset and skillset can also be useful in helping staff to "work well with" the challenges inherent in their roles.

Research into ACT and staff wellbeing

Flaxman et al. (2013) present a helpful summary of research demonstrating links between psychological flexibility and a broad range of employee and organisational outcomes, including performance, absence rates, stress and ways of coping with role demands. This review follows a comprehensive and detailed "manual" for a brief ACT intervention with employees (e.g. three sessions), designed to be adaptable across work settings and to fit different purposes, such as improving general resilience or facilitating leadership development. It encompasses ACT content (both in session and between) on mindfulness, work to clarify values and translate them into action and work around defusion and acceptance.

In addition, there is a small but growing evidence base highlighting the benefits of ACT competencies specifically on psychological clinicians' self-care. For example, Luoma and Vilardaga (2013) found that a 2-day ACT workshop, with six follow-up telephone consultations, increased psychological flexibility in a small sample of psychotherapists, and that increased benefits in psychological flexibility in this telephone consultation group were associated with lower scores on measures of burnout. Pakenham (2017) reported positive effects of a group intervention teaching ACT techniques specifically for self-care to two cohorts of trainee clinical psychologists, and previous work with similar small cohorts has demonstrated correlations between ACT processes (such as acceptance, defusion, valued living) and adjustment outcomes such as distress and life satisfaction (Pakenham, 2015; Stafford-Brown & Pakenham, 2012).

Practising ACT as a clinician

ACT can provide a framework for conceptualising some of the struggles of undertaking psychological work in ABI settings, as well as offering skills to increase one's own psychological flexibility. In line with other third-wave approaches, ACT emphasises the importance of therapists themselves having experienced the skills they teach to clients, to deepen their knowledge, congruence with the model and credibility. In addition, it is well suited for use in occupational wellbeing, as a transdiagnostic model of human experience (rather than pathology or diagnosis). This brings both preventative as well as therapeutic opportunities. ACT can be compatible with work settings given its "here-and-now", practical and skills-based focus, which is translatable to many different contexts.

Essentially, all ACT ideas and exercises used in work with clients could be relevant to apply to ourselves and our colleagues, either in their original form or with adaptation specifically to consider work roles. Here, some brief ideas will be presented, which may be relevant as adaptations or additions to clinicians working in ABI settings.

Open up

Acknowledging and accepting struggle and self-doubt can allow us to behave and respond flexibly, in line with values. Both for ourselves and others, we can make space for recognising the personal impact of the work, for example through valuing time spent chatting about a tough session, actively reflecting on the sadness and challenge in the work and providing all staff with supervision spaces. Reflective groups, organisation level meetings (e.g. Schwartz Center Rounds; Maben et al., 2018) and team formulation discussions (e.g. Geach et al., 2018) are forums where this open culture may also be created. We can all strive to keep the "human" at the centre of our teams, avoiding the creation of professionalised spaces or team styles, which inadvertently reinforce experiential avoidance. Many ACT exercises around tuning in to (rather than suppressing) pain or struggle can be useful here (e.g. Harris, 2019). These could be adapted to consider the challenges of work roles, in reflective review or "live" in the moment.

Exercise: How would you describe to a stranger why your job is hard?

Notice moments in the day when difficult feelings and thoughts arise. Try to sit in the moment, or return to it when you can, and reflect for a short time. Perhaps write a statement, or keep a journal, which acknowledges the feelings and thoughts, and the fact that you continue to work, alongside them. Consider the following prompts:

- What are the challenges contained in these moments, for you as a human being?
- What difficult feelings do you carry around, whilst still continuing to do your best with the work?
- Why is this situation tricky for you as an individual? What values are being challenged?
- What values are most important to you personally, to guide you during these difficult times?

Reread the statement or spend a moment in gentle acknowledgement, giving yourself some compassion, either through self-talk (e.g. recognising the inherent challenges in the job) or with a physical gesture, like a hand on the heart, a cup of tea.

EXAMPLE RESPONSE

I feel tense, with an anxious flutter in my stomach. I met someone today whose life has been devastated by their brain injury. I witnessed huge, raw emotions and had the job of providing containment to them and their family, and afterwards to my colleague, who felt lost with how we could help them. I really tried to listen well, and then straight afterwards to smile in the coffee room at the team Christmas party! I'm worried about all the people I can't manage to see because of a waiting list, and I feel angry about admin tasks I have to do which feel much less important. I sometimes just don't know what to do. I can't ever do enough to make things better. But I do carry on, do my best, be kind where I can and continue with the juggle.

Exercise: What would it be like not to feel?

Imagine doing this psychological work as a robot, an avatar in human form, but with no feelings or thoughts, just processes which deliver content or instruction to clients. Picture this slick, brilliant yet emotionless algorithm going about your daily tasks. Consider the following prompts as you reflect:

- What would it be like for clients to receive psychological input from someone with no emotional reaction to the work?
- Why is your humanity useful? What do your reactions and feelings bring to your work and presence with people?
- When have you drawn on your personal reactions and feelings in your work, and how has it gone?
- What would be the risks or drawbacks of getting rid of your empathy and warmth, your doubts, very human flaws and vulnerabilities?

Write yourself a statement that validates your imperfect, messy humanity – your flaws and vulnerabilities (and is likely to touch upon your values at work).

EXAMPLE RESPONSE

I feel and think things about my work. I really do want to do my best to show people validation, give clear information and to help them adjust by listening or offering ideas. I believe that being warm and understanding is just as important as being technically adept or full of knowledge. But this is hard – the struggle I have is normal, and part of my humanity. I cannot afford not to feel. I feel pain, stress, doubt – all because I care. If I didn't care, I wouldn't feel these emotions. I accept them. I need them. My clients and colleagues need them too.

Many exercises from compassion-focused therapy (e.g. Kolts, 2016) also fit well with using ACT in relation to self-care; indeed this cross-pollination has been recognised and usefully presented by ACT authors (e.g. Harris, 2017b). For example, it could be useful to listen to "compassionate other" audio exercises from compassion-focused therapy websites (e.g. Gilbert, 2016), and use the image you generate as a "compassionate supervisor", who really knows you as a clinician, and genuinely offers acceptance and warmth to your struggle and your successes (e.g. Bell, 2015).

Defusion

In common with the people they support, clinicians will be vulnerable to being "hooked" by thoughts, especially those longer-term (often negative) stories carried around about ourselves, probably from earlier experiences. Many ACT defusion exercises are likely to be useful with our own "hooks" (e.g. see Harris, 2019) – such as thanking one's mind, noticing common or repetitive "stories" and labelling them as such, or using guided practice such as "leaves on a stream" meditations.

It can be helpful to access accounts of other therapists' internal worlds, to help defuse from our own. For example, Colodro and Oliver (2018) shared their own versions of self-critical thoughts which "hook" them as individuals when in challenging therapeutic situations in a helpful e-book about therapist self-care. The personal tone of this was helpful in normalising the commonality and impact of the therapist's own internal world, from an ACT perspective. Russ Harris was interviewed on a podcast for newly qualified psychologists specifically on the subject of his own self-doubt (Harris, 2017a), illustrating the pervasiveness of struggle in therapeutic work, even for someone so influential in the development and dissemination of ACT ideas.

Exercise: Passengers on a therapist's bus

Think of a situation when your sense of confidence or competence at work has been shaken recently. Better still, observe this live, after a difficult session or meeting, or any time you find yourself being "hooked" by difficult internal experiences, or fusing with their messages.

The "passengers on a bus" metaphor, common in ACT resources (e.g. Hayes et al., 1999), offers a useful way to observe the thoughts that run through our mind. This adapted version includes questions that a clinician might ask themselves:

While you are "driving the bus" at work:

- What do your passengers shout? When are they loudest?
- What vulnerabilities do they go after?
- What impacts and consequences do the passengers have (intended or otherwise)?

- In what ways do the passengers help or hinder me in doing my job?
- What do the passengers tell me about my values? What good stuff are passengers trying to remind me of, in terms of values?
- Given that I know the passengers will show up, how do I want to drive (even while they are there)? What helps me to keep driving in the manner and direction I value?

Take a pen and paper. Design a driver's cab for your bus which will help you to keep driving (despite the passengers) in the direction and manner which you feel is best for you as a clinician working in ABI services, in line with your values. This might include physical features such as Perspex screens, radio systems, magic curtains, signs/statements, symbols or talismans, useful tools or equipment, a musical soundtrack or other audio, seats next to yours for a compassionate co-pilot – whatever will best allow you to keep driving as you want to.

Exercise: The role of self-doubt

When exploring the therapy outcomes of a large cohort of psychotherapists (Nissen-Lie et al., 2017), researchers found that the most effective therapists were those who had high levels of "professional self-doubt", especially if those therapists were able to feel generally kind and positive towards themselves more broadly. It is hypothesised that doubting oneself as a therapist actually helps, because it leads to self-review, critical engagement with broad perspectives and more constructive coping, such as sharing difficulties or seeking support.

Notice times when self-critical thoughts and feelings arise for you, and consider the following:

- What do these feelings and thoughts represent, which is good about you and your approach?
- What values do they connect you with?
- What would you be like if you never felt this self-doubt or self-criticism?
- What could be the risks of this?
- Would you want to be immune to the inevitable struggles which come from doing this important and meaningful work?
- Could you "thank your mind" in a positive way, without getting too involved with the content or "hooked"?

Be present

Our roles require an ability to stay available and connected to ourselves and others in the face of huge distress or challenge. ACT approaches often use mindfulness skills and other techniques to help people to be present, to notice feelings and thoughts in a broad way (without seeing them as facts), to allow people to maintain attention and sit with emotion without turning away (e.g. see Harris, 2019). A "body scan" between clinical sessions could be a way of bringing awareness back to the present, and "grounding techniques" can be a useful way for therapists to calm and soothe themselves in difficult moments, alongside offering containment to others. "Reflective practice", especially done live and in the moment, is a version of being present, and maintaining an overarching or "meta" awareness over and above "content". Making space to check in with colleagues regularly is important – even a simple and informal "How are you after that session?" or "What did that bring up for you?" can be invaluable in helping to notice difficult thoughts and feelings, defuse and bring someone's attention back to the here and now.

ACT suggests that seeing oneself as an observer, with natural and changing emotions and thoughts (rather than a fixed concept), can aid flexibility. Perhaps seeing oneself through the context of the work could be useful in addition, in giving perspective and aiding defusion – for example, making space to think about and reflect on what role we might need to take on within a therapeutic relationship, or what stance or style we might adopt with different clients in different situations.

Exercise: Recognising our common humanity

Picture all the psychological workers in ABI teams across your country, like an army, leaving their different homes each day to provide support and care to people who are experiencing pain, worry and disability. Imagine the feelings and thoughts of these people rising off them like continuous exhaust streams of multi-coloured vapour, which collect in the atmosphere above the earth. Imagine your own thoughts and feelings rising up off you every day, to join the collective cloud. Understand that they will always rise, like an ever-pumping air vent which may change colour or temperature, but which one would never want to block up or stop. They form part of a common humanity or impact, of which all workers in this field (including you) are a part.

Do what matters

According to ACT, connection with one's values, and committed action in the service of them, is the key to a vital and meaningful life – for clients and clinicians alike. Just as clarifying values can guide behaviour after a brain injury, it can help clinicians to manage inevitable tensions in pressured services, and the emotional impact of the work, as discussed above. Completing a formal values exercise in relation to our work roles can help us to understand ourselves, and why some situations challenge or invigorate us.

Exercise: Values cards

Using a deck of ACT values cards or a list of ACT values, consider the following questions:

- In this work, what are the core values that underlie how you strive to behave, go about your tasks and relate to clients?
- What does "great work" look like to you?
- How do you manifest these values, in both small and larger ways day to day?
- If a client or colleague wrote feedback about you, what values or ways of behaving would you want them to have noticed?
- What have you done in the past week which stems from any of these important values?
- When you notice suffering or pain in relation to our work, which of your precious values are under threat or are clashing?

Sharing results as a team can lead to cultures of shared endeavour, mutual respect, and understanding and celebration of difference.

Impact of the COVID-19 pandemic

While ABI settings have not been the "frontline" of COVID-19 pandemic care in the same way that accident and emergency and critical care services have been, disruptions to all public healthcare, and the overall increase in pressure through healthcare systems and society more generally, have certainly been felt by ABI healthcare staff, who have continued to work throughout all phases of the pandemic. Unlike other natural disasters, in which helpers are usually separate and distinct from the "helped", healthcare staff have juggled their own anxiety, bereavement and role pressures, whilst also trying to deliver work duties in unfamiliar circumstances. Cultural narratives around healthcare staff being "heroes" can anecdotally result in staff struggling to prioritise self-care and boundaries, due to guilt and competing life demands. Billings et al. (2020) examined what support healthcare professionals wanted through the early stages of the COVID-19 pandemic and identified the importance of a systemic approach based on consistency, peer support and ensuring that practical needs (e.g. for rest and food) were met. Stigma around seeking help was also identified as a barrier; it is important for services to ensure that the emphasis is not on individual staff to be "more resilient". The cultural, systemic and structural barriers to staff wellbeing are a key focus for intervention.

Increased stress for service users (from social isolation; delays and limitations in healthcare, rehabilitation and third-sector support; financial pressure; worries about health and more) inevitably impacts upon staff working in services. Work to support "adjustment" to an ABI can be hampered by disrupted services, and limited opportunity for service users to build new activities, roles and identities. The already high demand for psychological input has only increased, with a struggle to disentangle COVID-related distress from that more specifically related to ABI, in order to maintain service boundaries and keep workloads realistic. Service impacts (such as suspensions, faster discharges or disruptions to specialist care) result in staff finding it harder than ever to deliver care in line with their own expectations and values, and this "moral injury" (e.g. Williamson et al., 2020) has been widely recognised as a risk to staff emotional wellbeing.

Studies have shown associations between aspects of psychological flexibility and reduced distress during the COVID-19 pandemic in general populations (e.g. Dawson & Golijani-Moghaddam, 2020; Kroska et al., 2020). Research into the role of psychological flexibility, and ultimately the effectiveness of ACT interventions, in promoting wellbeing of healthcare staff in relation to the pandemic would be useful in the urgent task of supporting this depleted workforce to continue and to recover.

Among a plethora of psychological self-help resources available online throughout COVID-19, Russ Harris's *FACE COVID* e-book (2020) provides an accessible description of ACT processes highly relevant to staff (although not specifically aimed at them). The acronym (presented below) and descriptions provide a practical summary of how ACT might be implemented by staff (and others), validating distress as well as suggesting ways of coping and "living well" in the face of unprecedented struggle – a balance which is difficult though important to achieve with the healthcare workforce.

F = Focus on what's in your control
A = Acknowledge your thoughts and feelings
C = Come back into your body
E = Engage in what you're doing
C = Committed action
O = Opening up
V = Values
I = Identify resources
D = Disinfect and distance

Conclusion

Working in ABI services poses significant challenges for clinicians in terms of wellbeing, especially given the COVID-19 pandemic. An ACT framework can offer a guiding philosophy alongside practical techniques to help clinicians to accept the inevitable impact of the work, stay aware and engaged, and continue to be able to work according to their personal and professional values.

This psychological flexibility is likely to benefit healthcare workers as individuals, which in itself is likely to protect the healthcare workforce and enhance service user care.

Note

1 For the purposes of this chapter when we refer to clinicians and therapists, we are referring to all staff who work in acquired brain injury settings, whatever their role or professional background.

Suggested further reading

Colodro, H., & Oliver, J (2018). *ACT therapist guide to self care e-book* [pdf file]. https://contextualconsulting.co.uk/act-therapist-guide-to-self-care-e-book

Flaxman, P. E., Bond, F. W., & Livheim, F. (2013). *The mindful and effective employee – An acceptance and commitment therapy training manual for improving well-being and performance.* New Harbinger.

Harris, R. (2017, February 14th). Episode 40: Self doubt and fear of failure. *We all wear it differently* [audio podcast]. https://weallwearitdifferently.com/2017/02/actrussharris/

Harris, R. (2017). *Simple steps to self compassion* [pdf file]. http://thehappinesstrap.com/wp-content/uploads/2019/08/Simple-Steps-to-Self-Compassion-by-Dr.-Russ-Harris-2.pdf

Support the workers. Resources briefing notes for supporting staff during COVID-19. www.supporttheworkers.org/

References

Bell, T. (2015). *Compassionate supervisor creation* [audio file]. https://soundcloud.com/tobyn-bell/compassionate-supervisor-creation

Billings, J., Seif, N. A., Hegarty, S., Ondruskova, T., Soulios, E., Bloomfield, M., & Greene, T. (2020). What support do frontline workers want? A qualitative study of health and social care workers' experiences and views of psychosocial support during the COVID-19 pandemic. *BMJ* [preprint]. https://doi.org/10.1101/2020.11.05.20226522

Biron, M., & van Veldhoven, M. (2012). Emotional labour in service work: Psychological flexibility and emotional regulation. *Human Relations, 65*(10), 1259–1282. https://doi.org/10.1177/0018726712447832

Colodro, H., & Oliver, J. (2018). *ACT therapist guide to self care e-book* [pdf file]. https://contextualconsulting.co.uk/act-therapist-guide-to-self-care-e-book

Dawson, D. L., & Golijani-Moghaddam, N. (2020). COVID-19: Psychological flexibility, coping, mental health, and wellbeing in the UK during the pandemic. *Journal of Contextual Behavioral Science, 17*, 126–134. https://doi.org/10.1016/j.jcbs.2020.07.010

Flaxman, P. E., Bond, F. W., & Livheim, F. (2013). *The mindful and effective employee – An acceptance and commitment therapy training manual for improving well-being and performance.* New Harbinger.

Geach, N., Moghaddam, N. G., & De Boos, D. A. (2018). A systematic review of team formulation in clinical psychology practice: Definition, implementation and outcomes. *Psychology and Psychotherapy, 91*(2), 186–121. https://doi.org/10.1111/papt.12155

Gilbert, P. (2016). *Compassionate image and compassionate community* [audio file]. https://soundcloud.com/compassionatemind/compassionate-image-and-compassionate-community/s-oQoMN?in=compassionatemind/sets/compassionate-minds

Harris, R. (2017a, February 14). Episode 40: Self doubt and fear of failure. *We all wear it differently* [audio podcast]. https://weallwearitdifferently.com/2017/02/actrussharris/

Harris, R. (2017b). *Simple steps to self compassion* [pdf file]. http://thehappinesstrap.com/wp-content/uploads/2019/08/Simple-Steps-to-Self-Compassion-by-Dr.-Russ-Harris-2.pdf

Harris, R. (2019). *ACT made simple* (2nd ed.). New Harbinger.

Harris, R. (2020). FACE COVID – How to respond effectively to the Corona crisis [pdf file]. www.actmindfully.com.au/wp-content/uploads/2020/03/FACE-COVID-eBook-by-Russ-Harris-March-2020.pdf

Hayes, S. C., Strosahl, K. D., & Wilson, K. W. (1999). *Acceptance and commitment therapy: An experiential approach to behaviour change.* Guilford Press.

Kolts, R. L. (2016). *CFT made simple: A clinician's guide to practicing compassion-focused therapy.* New Harbinger.

Kroska, E. B., Roche, A. I., Adamowicz, J. L., & Stagnall, M. S. (2020). Psychological flexibility in the context of COVID-19 adversity: Associations with distress. *Journal of Contextual Behavioral Science, 18*, 28–33. https://doi.org/10.1016/j.jcbs.2020.07.011

Luoma, J. B., & Vilardaga, J. P. (2013). Improving therapist psychological flexibility while training acceptance and commitment therapy: A pilot study. *Cognitive Behaviour Therapy, 42*(1), 1–8. https://doi.org/10.1080/16506073.2012.701662

Maben, J., Taylor, C., Dawson, J., Leamy, M., McCarthy, I., Reynolds, E., Ross, S., Shuldham, C., Bennett, L., & Foot, C. (2018). A realist informed mixed-methods evaluation of Schwartz Center Rounds in England. *Health Services & Delivery Research, 6*(37), 1–260. https://doi.org/10.3310/hsdr06370

Nissen-Lie, H. A., Rønnestad, M. H., Høglend, P. A., Havik, O. E., Solbakken, O. A., Stiles, T. C., & Monsen, J. T. (2017). Love yourself as a person, doubt yourself as a therapist? *Clinical Psychology and Psychotherapy, 24*(1), 48–60. https://doi.org/10.1002/cpp.1977

Pakenham, K. I. (2015). Investigation of the utility of the acceptance and commitment therapy (ACT). Framework for fostering self-care in clinical psychology trainees. *Training and Education in Professional Psychology, 9*(2), 144–152. https://doi.org/10.1037/tep0000074

Pakenham, K. I. (2017). Training in acceptance and commitment therapy fosters self-care in clinical psychology trainees. *Clinical Psychologist, 21*, 186–194. https://doi.org/10.1111/cp.12062

Stafford-Brown, J., & Pakenham, K. I. (2012). The effectiveness of an ACT informed intervention for managing stress and improving therapist qualities in clinical psychology trainees. *Journal of Clinical Psychology, 68*(6), 592–513. https://doi.org/10.1002/jclp.21844

Williamson, V., Murphy, D., & Greenberg, N. (2020). COVID-19 and experiences of moral injury in frontline key workers. *Occupational Medicine, 70,* 317–319. https://doi.org/10.1093/occmed/kqaa052

Chapter 16

Future directions

Abigail Methley and Will Curvis

As the wealth of clinical experiences shared in this book shows, now is an exciting time for the application of acceptance and commitment therapy (ACT) within neurorehabilitation and neuropsychology settings. Whilst the clinical relevance of ACT within a range of neurorehabilitation settings is clear, further research to evidence this is key. Capturing further information on an individual level such as case studies and single-case experimental designs, through to larger cohort and longitudinal studies, will assess the effectiveness, efficacy and economical feasibility of this approach, compared to existing approaches and treatment as usual.

Van Heugten (2017) highlights the importance of valid and systematic outcome measures for measuring prognosis and outcomes. Appropriate measurement tools are vital in supporting rigorous analysis of therapeutic effectiveness and comparison across studies, providing necessary information for researchers, clinicians, managers, policy makers, patients and families. A broad range of measures exist assessing values across specific life domains, including the perceived importance of values and success in living consistently with values (see Reilly et al., 2019 for a systematic review). The format of some of these measures may need adapting for people with more severe cognitive impairments (e.g. the bull's-eye values survey, Lundgren et al. 2012, and measures using Likert scales).

Measures specifically designed and validated for brain injury populations include the Acceptance and Action Questionnaire – Acquired Brain Injury (AAQ-ABI), which measures psychological flexibility about the thoughts and feelings related to the brain injury (Whiting et al., 2015). Other measures not developed for people with brain injuries have also been used with these samples (Pais Hons et al., 2019; Rauwenhoff et al., 2019; Sander et al., 2020; Whiting et al., 2020). The Psychological Flexibility Questionnaire for People with Intellectual Disabilities (PFQ-ID) provides an adapted and accessible outcome measure which correlates highly with mainstream measures and shows good internal consistency (Oliver et al., 2019). Reilly et al. (2018) highlight the need for more international and non-Western measures, with culturally appropriate validation studies.

DOI: 10.4324/9781003024408-19

The convergence between ACT principles and an established neuro-psychological rehabilitation model has been presented (Chapter 3). Further research could explore how significant mechanisms within ACT, including experiential avoidance, psychological flexibility, ability to stay mindful, fit with established outcomes within traditional neuropsychological rehabilitation models to further conceptual understanding within applied settings. Innovative technological methods could offer an improved ability to measure the impact of ACT on outcomes such as awareness of difficulties in real time, rather than in retrospective self-report measures with their inherent biases.

Adapting ACT: Next steps

The personal experiences of Harriet, Paul and Holly provide valuable insights into why ACT may be relevant to people living with brain injury and their families. It is important that both qualitative and quantitative research is used to guide the practice and training of healthcare professionals in this field.

The majority of literature on ACT is for people with neurotypical communicative and cognitive functioning. This book has highlighted how ACT can be adapted to an individual's cognitive and communicative level, across the lifespan, by incorporating adaptations for both chronological age and life stage, and physical, cognitive or communication impairments (e.g. in the presence of severe brain injury). Through multidisciplinary practice and evaluation of these practices, we can ensure access to ACT-based approaches for a broad range of clients, even where there may have been initial therapeutic nihilism about their ability to engage in a "talking therapy".

Although we did not cover every kind of neurological condition, we hope that this book has offered a starting point for clinicians and researchers alike. We hope that some of the principles are applicable to a range of settings beyond brain injury and across the lifespan, such as services supporting people with dementia, intellectual disabilities or severe mental health problems. The transdiagnostic nature of the mechanisms targeted in ACT may also increase the feasibility of access to group treatment for people with a variety of diagnoses, including rarer neurological conditions. Whilst these conditions may be rare in terms of their individual prevalence, there are over 150,000 people living with rare neurological conditions in England alone (The Neurological Alliance, 2020), suggesting a cumulative need for transdiagnostic intervention that may be masked by a condition-specific focus. ACT may also give a message of therapeutic hope to staff members in more generalist services by providing a framework for intervention where physical symptoms are unlikely to change.

Neuropsychological populations benefit from digital scaffolding. Mobile apps which remind people of ACT strategies could be beneficial. Commonly available apps include ACT companion and ACT iCoach, with other examples present in the literature (Gentili et al., 2020; Kaipainen et al., 2017;

Kroska et al., 2020; Levin et al., 2017; Mattila et al., 2016; Trompetter et al., 2015) which could potentially be adapted and validated with people with brain injuries. The use of virtual and augmented reality is also developing in neurorehabilitation (Riva et al., 2020) and may provide novel access to exercises for developing ACT-based skills, such as completing challenging tasks to decrease avoidance or better understand values. These methods could be used to support values-based exposure for psychosocial goals including discharge planning, return to work and mental health support.

Systemic thinking: Next steps

It may not be initially clear how ACT principles could benefit people unable to engage in therapy directly and so the value of using ACT to indirectly improve support is presented using the clinical example of prolonged disorders of consciousness. This theme resonates across settings by showing how to support families and care teams of people with many different clinical conditions. Whilst there is a developing body of research on supporting carers using ACT interventions (Han et al., 2021), there is a great need for further research within neuropsychology populations.

ACT has a growing body of evidence on changing staff practice. The ethos of ACT is such that it does not require lengthy or prohibitively expensive formal training. Whilst caveats of course exist regarding the need for ethical, competent and appropriately supervised practice, where these are met ACT can provide an interactional framework for both qualified and pre-qualified professionals within health, social, forensic and education settings. In addition, it may prove a particularly useful model in services where conflict between professionals and service users is common, due to its ability to get underneath judgement-based or diagnostic-based discussions and focus instead on the utility of current approaches for that individual (similar to motivational interviewing approaches).

It would be beneficial to explore the ACT core competency self-rating form (items taken from Hayes & Strosahl, 2004) within neuropsychology settings to explore how the points apply and how best to provide supervision that enables the provision of ACT within a neuropsychological framework. The Y-Shaped model has also been used as a tool for supervision of clinical practice in neurorehabilitation settings (F. Gracey, personal communication, 25 March 2021) especially where psychological processes are significant for the rehabilitation professional, for example where they experience a parallel process of discrepancy from "ideal practitioner" within the pulls of the therapeutic process. Supervision can provide a parallel safe space in which the practitioner can explore their own identity-related drives in practice, and at the same time gain some experiential insights into aspects of their client's experience.

ACT approaches for supporting staff are now well established. Given the emotive nature of neurorehabilitation settings and the rare ethical decisions often faced, it would be beneficial to evaluate interventions within these settings to establish if any adaptations are required or whether they can be applied as is. This textbook was completed during the COVID-19 pandemic when ACT provided a framework for supporting individuals and communities in tolerating uncertainty and processing their individual and cumulative grief.

The potential for ACT to be applied to wider systems has been presented. Further conceptual and applied research could examine how ACT principles could be used to understand health services research topics including access to care, barriers and enablers to service use and both service user and healthcare professional decision making, based on personal and professional values.

References

Gentili, C., Zetterqvist, V., Rickardsson, J., Holmström, L., Simons, L. E., & Wicksell, R. K. (2020). ACTsmart – Development and feasibility of digital acceptance and commitment therapy for adults with chronic pain. *NPJ Digital Medicine, 3*, 20. https://doi.org/10.1038/s41746-020-0228-4

Gracey, F. *Personal communication*, 25 March 2021.

Han, A., Yuen, H. K., & Jenkins, J. (2021). Acceptance and commitment therapy for family caregivers: A systematic review and meta-analysis. *Journal of Health Psychology, 26*(1), 82–102. https://doi.org/10.1177/1359105320941217

Hayes, S. C., & Strosahl, K. D. (Eds.). (2004). *A practical guide to acceptance and commitment therapy*. Springer-Verlag.

Kaipainen, K., Välkkynen, P., & Kilkku, N. (2017). Applicability of acceptance and commitment therapy-based mobile app in depression nursing. *Translational Behavioral Medicine, 7*(2), 242–253. https://doi.org/10.1007/s13142-016-0451-3

Kroska, E. B., Hoel, S., Victory, A., Murphy, S. A., McInnis, M. G., Stowe, Z. N., & Cochran, A. (2020). Optimizing an acceptance and commitment therapy microintervention via a mobile app with two cohorts: Protocol for micro-randomized trials. *JMIR Research Protocols, 9*(9), e17086. https://doi.org/10.2196/17086

Levin, M. E., Haeger, J., Pierce, B., & Cruz, R. A. (2017). Evaluating an adjunctive mobile app to enhance psychological flexibility in acceptance and commitment therapy. *Behavior Modification, 41*(6), 846–867. https://doi.org/10.1177/0145445517719661

Lundgren, T., Luoma, J. B., Dahl, J., Strosahl, K., & Melin, L. (2012). The Bull's-Eye Values Survey: A psychometric evaluation. *Cognitive and Behavioral Practice, 19*(4), 518–526. https://doi.org/10.1016/j.cbpra.2012.01.004

Mattila, E., Lappalainen, R., Välkkynen, P., Sairanen, E., Lappalainen, P., Karhunen, L., Peuhkuri, K., Korpela, R., Kolehmainen, M., & Ermes, M. (2016). Usage and dose response of a mobile acceptance and commitment therapy app: Secondary analysis of the intervention arm of a randomized controlled trial. *JMIR Mhealth and Uhealth, 4*(3), e90. https://doi.org/10.2196/mhealth.5241

Oliver, M., Selman, M., Thomson, M., Brice, S., Long, R., & Forshaw, N. (2019). ACBS World Conference 17, World Conference, Dublin Ireland, 27–30th June 2019.

Pais Hons, C., Ponsford, J. L., Gould, K. R., & Wong, D. (2019). Role of valued living and associations with functional outcome following traumatic brain injury.

Neuropsychological Rehabilitation, 29(4), 626–637. https://doi.org/10.1080/09602011.2017.1313745

Rauwenhoff, J., Peeters, F., Bol, Y., & Van Heugten, C. (2019). The BrainACT study: Acceptance and commitment therapy for depressive and anxiety symptoms following acquired brain injury: Study protocol for a randomized controlled trial. *Trials, 20*, 773. https://doi.org/10.1186/s13063-019-3952-9

Reilly, E. D., Ritzert, T. R., Scoglio, A. A. J., Mote, J., Fukuda, S. D., Ahern, M. E., & Kelly, M. M. (2019). A systematic review of values measures in acceptance and commitment therapy research. *Journal of Contextual Behavioral Science, 12*, 290–304. https://doi.org/10.1016/j.jcbs.2018.10.004

Riva, G., Mancuso, V., Cavedoni, S., & Stramba-Badiale, C. (2020) Virtual reality in neurorehabilitation: A review of its effects on multiple cognitive domains. *Expert Review of Medical Devices, 17*(10), 1035–1061. https://doi.org/10.1080/17434440.2020.1825939

Sander, A. M., Clark, A. N., Arciniegas, D. B., Tran, K., Leon-Novelo, L., Ngan, E., Bogaards, J., Sherer, M., & Walser, R. (2020). A randomized controlled trial of acceptance and commitment therapy for psychological distress among persons with traumatic brain injury. *Neuropsychological Rehabilitation*, 31(7), 1105–1129. https://doi.org/10.1080/09602011.2020.1762670

The Neurological Alliance. (2020). *Out of the shadows: What needs to change for people with rare neurological conditions*. www.neural.org.uk/wp-content/uploads/2020/11/neurological-alliance-out-of-the-shadows-2020.pdf

Trompetter, H. R., Bohlmeijer, E. T., Veehof, M. M., & Schreurs, K. M. G. (2015). Internet-based guided self-help intervention for chronic pain based on acceptance and commitment therapy: A randomized controlled trial. *Journal of Behavioral Medicine, 38*, 66–80. https://doi.org/10.1007/s10865-014-9579-0

Van Heugten, C. M. (2017). Outcome measures. In B.A. Wilson, J. Winegardner, C.M. van Heugten, & T. Ownsworth (Eds.), *Neuropsychological rehabilitation: The international handbook* (pp. 537–546). Routledge.

Whiting, D., Deane, F., Ciarrochi, J., McLeod, H. J., & Simpson, G. K. (2015). Validating measures of psychological flexibility in a population with acquired brain injury. *Psychological Assessment*, 27(2), 415–423. https://doi.org/10.1037/pas0000050

Whiting, D., Deane, F., McLeod, H., Ciarrochi, J., & Simpson, G. (2020). Can acceptance and commitment therapy facilitate psychological adjustment after a severe traumatic brain injury? A pilot randomized controlled trial. *Neuropsychological Rehabilitation*, 30(7), 1348–1371. https://doi.org/10.1080/09602011.2019.1583582

Contributors

Dr Miriam Alonso Fernández is an Associate Professor in the Department of Psychology at the Universidad Rey Juan Carlos, Madrid, Spain. She studies psychological approaches to healthy ageing, dementia caregiving and chronic pain in older people. She has published work integrating the use of modern cognitive-behavioural therapy approaches with theoretical perspectives from geropsychology (selection, optimisation and compensation theory).

Dr Jo Black works as a Clinical Psychologist in a community neurorehabilitation service in the North West of England, delivering psychological assessment and intervention to adults (and their families) with a wide range of neurological conditions and acquired brain injuries, and working with team colleagues from a range of professional backgrounds. As a Clinical Tutor on the Doctorate in Clinical Psychology programme at Lancaster University, she is interested in the training and development of psychologists and other health professionals and in how we can remain compassionate, reflective and resilient clinicians in challenging roles and services.

Dr Ndidi Boakye is a Consultant Clinical Neuropsychologist at Guy's and St Thomas' NHS Trust, UK. She is also a Consultant Clinical Neuropsychologist and Lead Psychologist for Couples and Family Work in Brain Injury at the Wolfson Neurorehabilitation Centre at Queen Mary's Hospital at Roehampton, St George's University Hospitals Trust, UK. Dr Boakye has a special interest in working in cognitive rehabilitation, with distressed couples, adjustment issues, vocational rehabilitation, issues of diversity, supervision and process issues in team working. Her main therapy modalities include cognitive-behavioural therapy, systemic and psychodynamic psychotherapy.

Dr Emma Cameron is a Specialist Clinical Psychologist in the NHS working in a neuropsychology setting with people with acquired brain injuries and rare neurological conditions, where people often present with comorbid long-term physical health problems, substance misuse and pain. Emma became interested in the use of third-wave cognitive-behavioural therapies during her clinical psychology training and after qualifying in 2015 went on to complete further specialist training in ACT. She has worked across acute inpatient hospital settings and inpatient neurorehabilitation, through to outpatient and community settings.

Dr Will Curvis is a Senior Clinical Psychologist and has worked mainly in acute inpatient physical health and neuropsychology services with people with long-term physical health problems, pain problems or neurological conditions, across the North West of England. He also works as a Clinical Tutor for the Doctorate in Clinical Psychology programme at Lancaster University, UK.

Dr Audrey Daisley is a Consultant Clinical Neuropsychologist based in Oxford, UK. She specialises in and is passionate about working with families affected by neurological illness and injury. She divides her time between working in private practice and the NHS, offering creative and innovative family-focused services; her area of particular expertise is working with children who have a parent with a brain injury. Audrey has shared her work extensively through teaching, training, invited conference presentations and research. She is the co-author of several books, book chapters and peer-reviewed journal papers focused on family issues in neurorehabilitation.

Dr David T. Gillanders is a Senior Lecturer and Head of Clinical and Health Psychology at the University of Edinburgh. He is a Fellow of the Association for Contextual Behavioural Science, a peer-reviewed ACT trainer and has extensive experience in clinical practice of using ACT to help people with persistent health conditions, including neurological illness. His research programme has pursued work on basic measurement in ACT, understanding relationships between psychological flexibility and health as well as intervention studies of ACT in persistent health problems.

Dr Sarah Gillanders is a Consultant Clinical Neuropsychologist, an Associate Fellow of the British Psychological Society and a Full Member of the British Psychological Society Division of Neuropsychology. She has worked extensively in NHS services for people with a range of neurological conditions, including acquired brain injury and progressive conditions. She currently works in independent practice, undertaking assessment, rehabilitation and psychological therapies, with a broad range of neuropsychological presentations.

Dr Fergus Gracey is Clinical Associate Professor of Clinical Psychology in the Department of Clinical Psychology and Psychological Therapy at University of East Anglia, UK. He also has an honorary role as Consultant

Clinical Neuropsychologist with the Cambridge Centre for Paediatric Neuropsychological Rehabilitation in Cambridgeshire, UK. Previously Fergus was lead psychologist at the Oliver Zangwill Centre, Ely, UK. He completed his PhD on executive functions in everyday life following brain injury in 2019 and researches and writes on the topic of psychological adaptation to life following acquired brain injury.

Dr Victoria Gray is a Consultant Clinical Psychologist and Lead for the Clinical Health Psychology department at Alder Hey Children's NHS Foundation Trust in Liverpool, UK. Since qualifying as a Clinical Psychologist in 2003 her work has focused on supporting young people with acquired brain injury and their families through clinical and neuro-psychological assessment and intervention. She holds an active research portfolio and provides teaching to local Doctorate in Clinical Psychology courses.

Holly suffered a brain injury as a result of a car hitting her at 52 mph when she was a pedestrian. "I felt compelled to write about my recovery in the hope people like me and academics alike could learn from my lived experience. Without Dr Curvis' support and guidance I would never have realised the power of expressing myself in words. I am indebted to his, and the medical profession's, understanding of brain injury and healing routes to rehabilitation. Without them I wouldn't have found myself a new acceptable identity."

Harriet Holmes is an Assistant Psychologist working in neurodisability services. She contributed to this book to reflect on her own experiences following her mother's brain injury.

Dr Rosco Kasujja is a Clinical Psychologist based in Uganda. He is currently the Head of Department of Mental Health at the School of Psychology at Makere University, Uganda. Dr Rosco is interested in the scaling up of mental health in Uganda and has been one of the individuals rolling out ACT to both non-specialists and students at Makerere University. His main therapy modalities include ACT, interpersonal psychotherapy, systemic and psychodynamic psychotherapy.

Dr Lorraine King is a Consultant Clinical Neuropsychologist who has worked within NHS neuropsychology and neurorehabilitation services since qualifying as a clinical psychologist in 2005. She currently leads various strands of the clinical neuropsychology service with North Staffordshire Combined Healthcare NHS Trust, UK. Lorraine has clinical and research interests in traumatic brain injury, using ACT in neurological populations and patient experience of neuropsychological assessment. Lorraine is passionate about delivering high-quality services, enjoys teaching and supervising many promising newcomers to the field and is most thankful she discovered ACT for the help and insights it offers both to her clients, and for her own life.

Dr Mary King is a Clinical Psychologist working in the NHS. She has worked within community, outpatient and inpatient rehabilitation services for individuals with brain injuries, neurological conditions and physical health problems. Dr King currently works within the specialist Non-Epileptic Attack Disorder (NEAD) service at the Clinical Neuropsychology Department, Salford Royal NHS Foundation Trust, Greater Manchester, UK.

Dr Rebecca Large is a Clinical Psychologist in the NHS and is currently employed by the Community Neurological Rehabilitation Service in Aneurin Bevan University Health Board, UK. She is the Psychology Lead for the Acquired Brain Injury team within this service. She has particular interests in ACT and its applications within brain injury and stroke contexts, and actively contributes to the current evidence base. She has published research on stroke survivors' experiences of ACT and processes associated with post-stroke adjustment, and is currently running a randomised waitlist control study of ACT in acquired brain injury.

Dr Abigail Methley is a Senior Clinical Psychologist within an NHS neuro-psychology service in addition to independent practice. Since qualifying she has gained further experience of working with people with a range of neurological and mental health conditions, supporting them, their families and multidisciplinary care teams within acute, outpatient and community settings. She has expertise in supporting people who have experienced traumatic events and is a qualified eye movement desensi-tisation and reprocessing (EMDR) therapist.

Nadine Mirza is a Postgraduate Researcher with the Centre for Primary Care and Health Services Research at the University of Manchester, UK. She leads the Dementia in Ethnic Minorities (DOME) project. She has a back-ground in Psychology and an MPhil in primary care mental health with a focus on culturally sensitive cognitive testing. This culminated in her interest in ethnicity and dementia and has led to working towards a PhD focused on ethnic minorities' access of dementia services and the diag-nostic process, and also undertaking research on ethnic minorities' access of neuropsychological services. She is currently a committee member and assistant editor for the British Psychological Society's Minorities' Group.

Professor Reg Morris currently works for the Universities of Plymouth and Cardiff, UK. He is a Clinical Psychologist and has been a Programme Director for Doctorate in Clinical Psychology training since 2001. Since 1996 he has worked in NHS stroke services and on improving third-sector care in the Stroke Association and Bristol After Stroke. He co-authored the revised British Psychological Society Briefing Paper 19 on stroke and has published stroke articles on depression, anxiety, compliance with guidelines, carers, young strokes, experiences in services and ethnicity. He is a co-author of *Psychological Management of Stroke* (2012) and *Rebuilding Your Life After Stroke* (2017), an ACT-based self-help book for people who have experienced stroke.

Dr Mark A. Oliver is a Clinical Psychologist working with the Learning Disabilities Community Treatment Team in Northumberland. He has special interests in ACT, Relational Frame Theory, applied behaviour analysis and positive behavioural support. He seeks to combine these to help people whose mental health needs or presentations of challenging behaviour require bespoke adaptations.

Dr Ray Owen is a Consultant Clinical Psychologist and Health Psychologist with over 20 years' experience of working in physical health settings within the NHS. He has substantial experience of teaching and supervision in a wide range of contexts, both within the NHS and on a freelance basis. He is a Fellow of the Higher Education Academy, and an accredited facilitator in the national Advanced Communication Skills Programme for senior cancer practitioners. He is also an Association of Contextual Behavioural Science Peer Reviewed Trainer. Ray has taught extensively on ACT in physical health contexts and is the author of two successful self-help books published by Routledge, *Facing the Storm* (2011) and *Living with the Enemy* (2014), both of which were shortlisted for the British Medical Association Popular Medicine Book of the Year Award.

Dr Lindsay Prescott is a Clinical Psychologist working in a community stroke and neurorehabilitation service. She worked within brain injury rehabilitation services for several years prior to commencing clinical psychology training and has continued to broaden her experience within neuropsychology since. She completed her core and specialist final placements within clinical neuropsychology and conducted a doctoral thesis investigating psychological factors specific to mild traumatic brain injuries. Lindsay is keen to contribute to research in this area and is passionate about furthering her knowledge and application of ACT approaches within this context.

Dr Ché Rosebert is a Clinical Psychologist and Organisational Consultant with many years' experience of working with adults with complex needs and staff groups within the NHS, charity and private sectors. Ché is Director of External Relations for the Association of Clinical Psychologists UK. Most of Che's current work is within the field of homelessness and she is particularly keen on social justice, inclusion and learning from others.

Thomas Rozwaha is a final-year trainee Clinical Psychologist and doctoral student in clinical psychology at Lancaster University, UK. He currently works in a clinical health psychology service and has a particular interest in physical health and neuropsychology. Tom completed an MSc in molecular neuroscience before entering doctoral training. Since beginning clinical psychology training, he has worked in the neuropsychological assessment of both acute traumatic brain injury and degenerative conditions, and has used a variety of therapeutic approaches to support people with brain injuries, including ACT.

Dr Emily Smart is a Clinical Psychologist currently working in Pennine NHS Foundation Trust in Stockport, UK. She has experience working across acute neuropsychology and older people's services supporting people with a range of neurological and psychological difficulties and their families.

Dr Rachel Tams is a Consultant Clinical Neuropsychologist who specialises in working with individuals and families affected by neurological illness and injury. Based in Oxford, UK, she has over 25 years' experience of working in neurorehabilitation within the NHS and in private practice. Through this work Rachel has gained extensive experience of working with adults, families and carers affected by a wide range of neurological conditions, including brain injury. Throughout her clinical work Rachel has observed the many challenges faced by family members after their lives are affected by brain injury, the similarities and differences in their experiences post-injury and the resilience so often shown by families, and has found ACT to be a powerful way of working with those living with brain injury.

Dr Alistair J. Teager is a Consultant Clinical Neuropsychologist working at Salford Royal NHS Foundation Trust Hospital, Greater Manchester, UK. He is the clinical lead for neuropsychology input for acute neurorehabilitation and major trauma. Alistair does inpatient and out-patient work, and has research interests in emergency preparedness, major trauma, digitisation of clinical practice and prolonged disorders of consciousness.

Dr Victoria Teggart is a Clinical Neuropsychologist working in both NHS and private practice in Greater Manchester, UK. She has worked across a range of neuropsychological assessment and rehabilitation services since qualifying in 2006 and is currently working in stroke rehabilitation and neuropsychology in mental health. She has developed an interest in ACT over the past 5 years and applies this in her clinical work wherever possible.

Dr Cara Thompson is a Clinical Psychologist working in the NHS. Since qualifying in 2018 from Staffordshire University, UK, Cara has worked in inpatient neurorehabilitation services in Manchester and Liverpool, and a mental health neuropsychological assessment service. She also worked in hospital and outpatient neurorehabilitation settings both prior to and during her clinical training. She has a keen interest in ACT, having undertaken training in this approach, and she applies this flexibly to meet the needs of her clients, their families and the systems she works in.

Paul Twist is a 42-year-old stroke survivor who had a stroke at the age of 35. Paul wanted to contribute to this book to offer first-hand experiences as a brain injury survivor, with the hope that it might help health professionals to understand how things are from the perspective of someone who has experienced a brain injury.

Dr Katrina Vicentijevic is a Clinical Psychologist working clinically at Livability Icanho, a specialist acquired brain injury rehabilitation service in Suffolk, England. She is interested in how psychological models of formulation and intervention, including third-wave approaches, can support emotional adjustment and adaption post-brain injury. She completed her Clinical Psychology Doctoral thesis on mindfulness-based interventions and their effect on cognition and specific emotion processes in the context of acquired neurological conditions.

Dr Stephen Weatherhead is a Consultant Clinical Psychologist, Senior Academic Tutor with the Liverpool Clinical Psychology Programme and Co-Director of NeuroTriage. He is a father, brother, uncle, nephew and son (though his parents are both deceased). He had a difficult childhood, but with the help of many wonderful people has grown into a reasonably well-adjusted adult. He still has some struggles and is constantly learning more about himself and how he wants to be in the world. He believes the world is a good and beautiful place, and that if we hold true to the importance of community and connection, we will all continue to make the world a little bit better tomorrow than it was yesterday.

Professor Ingram Wright is a Consultant Paediatric Neuropsychologist and Head of Psychology Services at University Hospitals Bristol and Weston NHS Trust. He has worked as a Clinical Neuropsychologist at several tertiary neuroscience centres in the UK since qualifying as a Clinical Psychologist in 2000. Ingram was appointed inaugural Chair of the Faculty of Paediatric Neuropsychology in 2011. His clinical role involves assessment and intervention for children who have acquired brain injury. He uses ACT-based approaches to understand and support families and young people.

Index